A Western Horseman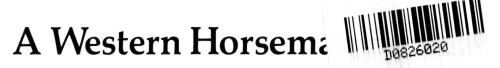

Colorado Springs, Colorado

HEALTH
PROBLEMS
OF THE HORSE

By Robert M. Miller

Edited by Gary Vorhes

HEALTH PROBLEMS
OF THE HORSE

Published by
The Western Horseman, Inc.

3850 North Nevada Avenue
P.O. Box 7980
Colorado Springs, CO 80933-7980

Design, Typography, and Production
Western Horseman
Colorado Springs, Colorado

Cover photo
By Debby Miller

Printing
Williams Printing
Colorado Springs, Colorado

ISBN 0-911647-13-9

DEDICATION

To Dick Spencer
I have practiced veterinary medicine for more than 30 years.
Throughout this time, I kept up a second career as a writer
and cartoonist, started before I graduated from veterinary
school because Dick Spencer, then editor and later publisher
of *Western Horseman* magazine, saw value in my work. He
was the first to buy my cartoons and my writing, launching
an avocation that has been as fulfilling and as challenging as
veterinary practice, and which has complemented it
throughout my career. Thank you, Dick.

To Betty and Babe
The draft team I drove as a boy. I learned to ride on their
sweat-soaked backs, coming in from the fields. They were
the first horses I worked with, and my love for horses (and
mules) has never left me.

RMM

ROBERT M. MILLER

INTRODUCTION

This book was originally published in 1967. At that time an up-to-date book on horse health, written in layman's language, was not available to horse owners. A compilation of articles I had done for *Western Horseman* was, therefore, published by that magazine, to fill that need.

That book has been in need of revision because of the great advances in veterinary technology since it was published. The horse population of the United States has increased by millions since 1967. The horse, which was at that time a rather neglected species, is now the subject of great attention, many research projects, and abundant literature.

An accurate veterinary manual, written so that horse owners of varied backgrounds can understand it, is needed in every stable. In this book I have tried to explain the complexities of pathology, diagnosis, and therapeutics the way I have explained them to thousands of my clients. I have also tried to remove as much of the mystique, superstition, and folklore from equine medicine as possible. It was inevitable that primitive man should apply the same concepts of folk medicine and witch-doctoring to the horse as he applied to himself. There is no room for such unscientific methods in the late twentieth century. Equine medicine is an enlightened science.

CONTENTS

1 MANAGEMENT

Horse Psychology

Physicians know it's difficult to separate human medicine from human psychology, the science of the mind. The will to live, for example, has long been recognized as an important part of recovery from a physical ailment. As a practicing equine veterinarian, I think it's equally difficult to separate equine medicine from equine psychology. And I believe every good equine practitioner should be not only a good horse handler, but a good horse psychologist.

No other horseman—trainer, farrier, groom, nobody—has to handle such large numbers of horses under such unfavorable conditions; frequently the horses are injured and in pain. They are nearly always scared, and the vet is nearly always in a hurry as he performs frightening (to the animal) procedures: giving injections, passing stomach tubes, doing dentistry, performing rectal and vaginal examinations, suturing wounds, opening abscesses, delivering foals, etc. No worse set of circumstances exists for compatibility between horse and human; and thus the veterinarian, who may treat up to 100 horses a day, must become proficient at horse handling or he can't work effectively, and will suffer an excessive number of injuries.

I do feel that the use of tranquilizing drugs is justified to save the doctor's valuable time, and to allay the patient's fear. Drugs, however, can't be used on every horse presented to the veterinarian; and, in fact, only a small percentage of equine patients are tranquilized for treatment.

I worked with horses for many years and broke many colts before becoming a veterinarian. But nearly all that I know today about horse handling, I have learned during my years as an equine practitioner. Although many people work with horses, few, I believe, have any real understanding about the mind of the horse. I've seen force and sometimes brutality used where finesse could achieve far superior results with far less effort. For this reason, I'd like to share some important things I've learned about the mind of this beast—ancient servant of man.

Horses have extraordinary memories. They never forget a veterinarian once he has treated them, and can even recognize a doctor they have never seen before, probably by the odor of medications, his dress, his truck, and his equipment. The horse is far more intelligent than most horsemen are aware of, and learning to get along with horses is a never-ending interest to me. The techniques I use can be learned by anyone with an open mind; and with practice, a whole new area of horsemanship can unfold.

There are three facets to the horse's mind, which once understood, help us get along with him. These are: 1/ His instinctive timidity. 2/ His ability to put aside his fearful instinctive responses once he learns that a frightening stimulus is harmless. 3/ His ability to accept domination.

Timidity is the single most basic personality quality of the equine species, and this is the key to understanding horses, setting the foundation to what

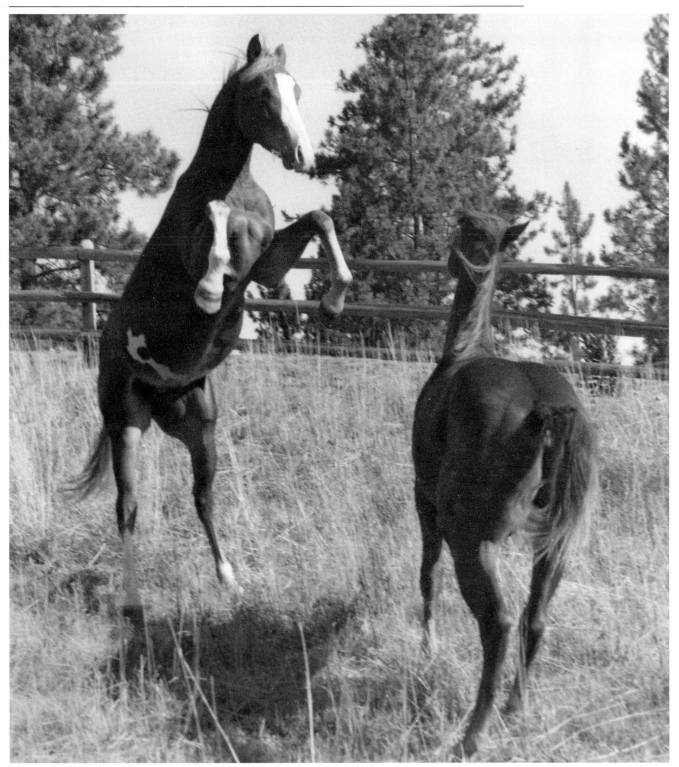

Photo by Russell Moray

follows. Horses are timid creatures . . . grazing animals whose instinctive reaction is to run from anything frightening. This is not to say that the horse is incapable of aggressive action or that some horses aren't mean. But the horse is basically fearful because in the primitive wild, fear and instant flight meant survival for this species.

In the course of evolution, every species of animal developed certain qualities to survive. Nature's law—survival of the fittest—ensured that these qualities were perpetuated. These qualities took an infinite variety of forms, including protective coloration, escape mechanisms (like speed and agility), anatomical weapons (like horns, fangs, or claws), and personality characteristics (like ferocity or, conversely, timidity and

The amazing thing is how adaptable the horse is to man's needs.

prompt flight). The antelope that ran too slowly didn't survive to reproduce its kind. The hawk with weak eyes died prematurely.

Inheritable variations became genetically fixed in a species by inbreeding. The first rhinoceros born with a horn on its nose was better able to stay alive and compete in the mating game than those without horns. It passed the ability to grow a horn to its progeny, and it wasn't long before all successful rhinos had horns. Then those with the longest and sharpest horns competed more successfully than those with shorter and duller horns.

The mechanism by which all these qualities are transmitted from generation to generation involves genes and chromosomes, fantastic structures within the body cells. Once a quality is genetically fixed within a species by natural selection, it is very difficult and often impossible to eliminate that quality from the species, even with many generations of artificial selection. Our domestic animals, like the horse, were established by artificial selection, in which man, rather than nature, determines which animals breed to which animals. However, all these animals, though slightly "modified" by man, came from the eons of natural selection—a horse is a horse by nature.

Let's use dogs as an example, before we take a closer look at the horse. In the wild state, dogs were hunting pack animals. All wild dogs (coyotes, wolves, jackals, dingoes, primeval wild dogs, etc.) have certain evolved characteristics in common that aid in their hunting existence. All have erect ears; pointed muzzles; sharp teeth; medium-length coats; brushy tails; keen eyes; an excellent sense of smell; long, slender bodies; and long, thin legs. Man domesticated the dog, and by artificial selection, grossly changed the physical appearance of certain strains within the species. Certainly a Basset hound, Pekingese, Saint Bernard, bulldog, or a Dalmation bears little resemblance to a wild dog. Yet, they are all dogs. They are all of one species.

Although man has changed the breeds physically to suit his needs or desires, there are certain mechanisms of survival, which we call instincts, that have

not changed in domestic dogs. They still lift their legs and urinate on trees to mark their hunting territory, though they no longer hunt. They still circle around to crush down the grass before they lie down, even though there is no grass and they sleep on the living room rug. Dogs still have pack instincts, wagging their tails to signal friendship to dogs or humans they recognize as a member of their pack. They bark at strangers whom they regard as competitors invading their hunting territory, and show great loyalty to their masters, whom they regard as leader of the pack.

What I'm saying is, the dog has been physically distorted, sometimes grotesquely distorted from his wild state, and yet he's still a dog, still acts like a dog, and will crossbreed with other dogs. In the case of the horse, we've greatly modified the wild conformation of the primitive horse, but we haven't changed him nearly as drastically as we have the dog.

In the primitive state, the horse evolved to survive on the open, grassy plains. This is his most natural environment. The primitive horse was small, tough, and colored to blend with the background. He had strong jaws and teeth to help him graze when the grass was dry and sparse. His natural enemies were the big carnivores: the big cats, the wolf, the bear. Even as today the zebra's natural enemy is the lion, so were the saber-toothed tiger and the other great cats the early horse's most feared predators.

The horse evolved to survive these enemies by developing a keen sense of hearing and smell. His eyes are special, and totally unlike ours. Each eye sees a separate picture. While the horse sees primarily in black and white, not full color, his eyes are set laterally on the sides of his head so that with a slight turn of his neck he can see behind himself, commanding a full view of the surrounding plain. Although the horse has difficulty distinguishing objects at any distance, what his eyes can do is pick up motion. A horse can detect the flicker of a leaf across a canyon, a movement invisible to his rider. And the horse has a reflector within his eye—the tapetum lucidum—that glows in the dark, and gives him far better night vision than man's. Remember, the horse stayed alive by detecting movement and running away.

Those horses that ran too slowly or stopped running too soon became a meal for a cat. And as time passed, the instincts became fixed—run when frightened. Run when a twig snaps, when a suspicious odor assails the nose, when something moves in the grass. Run when you unexpectedly walk upon a dark cave or a hole in the ground—caves hold bad things for horses. Run if any other horse runs; run blindly and wildly away from the fear and possible danger.

Horses have retained these instincts. Every foal is born with them; these behavioral traits are in the genes. Horses don't shy and run away, spook and charge through fences because of stupidity; this is nature's wisdom. After all, the horse wasn't designed to live in stalls or small paddocks surrounded by fences; horses are creatures of the open country, and anyone who handles horses should remember the fearful flight reaction.

It is a tribute to man's ingenuity that he found this unique animal, tamed him, and communicated with him, befriended him, and established a partnership with him. And it is the horse's versatility and his distinct psychological makeup that enabled man, thousands of years ago, to domesticate the horse and change the course of human history. A horse is naturally timid; but because his mind also has the ability to put aside his fearful instinctive responses once he learns that a frightening stimulus is harmless, and because he also accepts domination, he has been man's most loyal servant through the years.

The amazing thing is how adaptable the horse is to man's needs. We ask horses to do things that totally violate their natural instincts. We ask horses to tolerate riders carrying flapping flags, swinging ropes, discharging firearms, and blowing bugles. Horses jump 6½-foot fences, cross narrow bridges, load into dark and vibrating trailers, carry riders with flowing robes. They work cattle, buffalo, even geese; they carry dead cougars on their backs, charge down near-vertical mountainsides, and swim rivers. Horses tolerate fireworks, parades, ocean surf, motorcycles, and cement mixers roaring by. They accept New York City traffic, rampaging rioters, roaring cannons, and charging bulls. All are contrary to the horse's instinct for survival.

And when the horse fails man, it is usually man's fault. When horses fail to accomplish man's desires, injure man, or injure themselves, man is usually to blame. Most of the trouble we have with horses is caused by that fear within them. If a horse is not handled properly, fear may cause him to resort to such behavior as striking, rearing, kicking, or shying. In time, these may become habitual responses.

Such responses can be avoided with proper training; in fact, they can even be corrected in most cases, though it is always easier to prevent bad habits than it is to cure them. Most bad habits are man-made, but please understand that I'm not advocating that horses be spoiled and babied, as I'll point out later. It *is* necessary to dominate the horse, to use force, and sometimes even to inflict pain. But nothing should be done to increase fear. Fear makes a horse unreasonable. The sole exception to this is the aggressive horse; the occasional horse that lacks fear and attacks a human needs to have some fear—or respect—put into him, but in the great majority of cases, the difficult horse is difficult because he's afraid, not because he lacks fear.

Thus far, we've discussed the role of fear as a horse's basic survival response. Now we're going to discuss the horse's ability to overcome fear by habituation. This is a psychologist's term and it means to get an animal accustomed to a given condition or experience through repetition. By repeatedly showing the horse that he won't be hurt by the flapping flag, for example, he will gradually lose his fear of the flag and come to ignore it.

A horse can be frightened through one or more of the sensory stimuli: tactile—sense of touch, auditory—hearing, visual—seeing, and olfactory—smelling. But a horse can overcome these fears by repeated exposure to whatever stimuli are frightening him, provided the stimuli aren't painful. If they are painful, then the horse's fearful reaction is justified in his mind, and he will become more fearful. But if the exposure is repeated, and

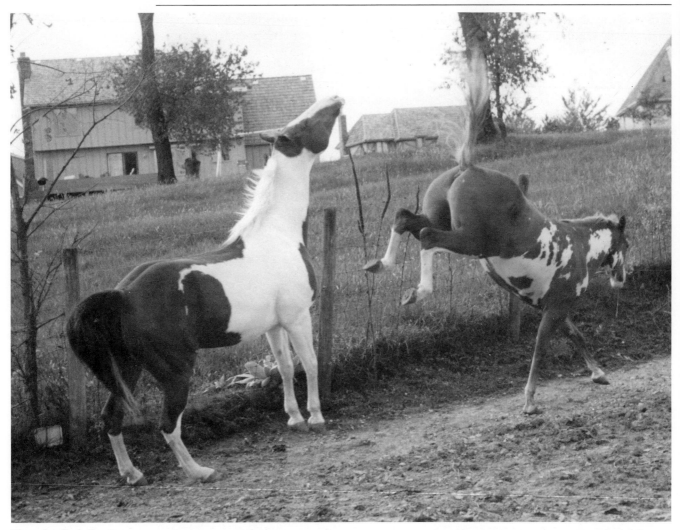

Photo by Carla Farris

repeated, and is never painful, the horse will sooner or later become habituated to it.

A common example of how this works occurs when we "sack out" a colt. We restrain the colt and then start waving a sack or blanket at him; he's terrified. He sees something, feels something, and hears something, and tries to get away, but can't because we've got him properly restrained, and have him under control in a small, enclosed space with a good halter and lead rope. With each wave of the sack he is increasingly frightened; and then sooner or later (it may take 30 seconds or maybe many minutes depending on the horse's disposition), he suddenly seems to realize that this frightening thing is not hurting him. He will start to quiet down, and if the sacking procedure is repeated constantly, the horse will finally ignore it. He is then, as we say, "broke to the sack." He has become habituated to this frightening stimulus so that it's no longer frightening to

him. The lesson will last a lifetime.

If the horse is somehow injured during the sacking process, if pain is inflicted, then his fear has become justified in his mind, and he might be afraid of flapping objects for the rest of his life. It's very important for the horseman to understand just what effect the sacking-out procedure has on the horse.

Another example. Say we're trying to train a horse for trail horse classes, and he's afraid of a green cowhide on the fence. What do we do? We hang one in the corral, or maybe put one on the ground and feed grain on it. What we're doing is habituating the horse to olfactory, visual, and tactile stimuli that are frightening. Once the horse realizes there is no basis to his fear, and that there's no pain inflicted, he is habituated. Horses overcome their fear of practically everything by habituation, and that's the reason an older and truly well-broke horse is unflappable.

Through habituation, foals should be

indoctrinated with the principle: "I must never touch a human, but any human can touch or handle me." Foals should be haltered, taught to lead, and then curried, brushed, petted, and scratched over every inch of their bodies. This includes the ears, the inside of the nostrils, the mouth, soles of the feet, under the tail, everywhere. Each new area touched may elicit a new fear response, but you should persist until the fear is gone. And fear will abate if you never hurt the foal. By the same token, though, don't allow foals to suck and nibble at your fingers or shirt buttons. Flick a foal's nose with your finger if he does this. Failure to do so might create a nipping horse.

The use of rhythmical stimuli in habituating a horse to many things is well recognized by horsemen, though they may never have stopped to analyze what they're doing. The rhythmical jingling of a halter by a horseman who's attempting to lightly restrain a horse, to make him stand still, is an example of what we're talking about. Skilled riders use rhythmical stimuli in communicating with a horse; for instance, the light quivering of the reins between the fingers can be used when you want to help calm a horse.

If we take a green horse and make a sudden hissing sound, it will terrify him. But if we repeatedly make that sound rhythmically, he will eventually stop jumping around, and will become habituated to it; if you persist long enough, he'll become nearly mesmerized by that sound. Old-time horsemen know this, and as they work around horses, they will make either a little whistling sound, or a little hissing sound, or maybe a little clucking sound, and they'll do it rhythmically.

When I'm breaking a horse to a thermometer, I don't just jam the thermometer into him and frighten him. I use rhythmical stimuli with my fingers, touching his hindquarters and gradually moving under the tail. When he's used to that, I gently rub him under the tail in the same rhythmical fashion, and finally he's ready for the thermometer. A similar procedure should be used in first bridling a horse. We don't just jam the bit into his mouth; we gently work it in, because if the horse is hurt at any time during our attempts at habituating, his

fear will only worsen. And this is why we get horses that are ear-shy, bridle-shy, or cinch-bound. All of the bad habits horses get come from reinforcing their natural fears, and failure to habituate them to frightening stimuli.

Next point: We can actually accelerate habituation by exposing the horse to repeated, rhythmic, *multiple* stimuli. When sacking a colt out, for example, instead of just using the sack, we can also use sounds, like the soothing whistling or hissing, or we can use a word, repeated over and over. Say we're teaching a young colt to be handled. We start brushing his legs for the first time and he's frightened, but as we rhythmically and gently brush the legs we say "easy, easy, easy," or "good boy, good boy, good boy." Or, a low whistle is what I like to use. By giving him multiple stimuli, two or three at a time, the habituation is reinforced. I can't explain why this happens, but it does speed up the habituation process.

The most common example I can use out of my own work is when I'm breaking a horse to a stomach tube. Passing a stomach tube up a horse's nose isn't painful, but it is very frightening to a horse. And if the horse has been handled roughly when being tubed in the past, and had a twitch roughly applied, then he's even more afraid, because his initial fear was reinforced. Please understand, I'm not opposed to twitches if they're used properly. But in breaking the horse to a stomach tube I simply start to scratch him on the face and somewhat simultaneously make little hissing sounds. And when he calms down and becomes habituated to that (in most horses, it takes from 30 to 60 seconds), I start moving toward the nostrils. Another 30 seconds or so and I can move my finger into the nostril.

He will react to that, but I gently keep making my little hissing, soothing noise, and simultaneously start to wiggle my finger inside the nostril, wiggling it rhythmically and in cadence with the noise. At the same time I'm using my other hand to scratch him elsewhere on the face. He's now getting three rhythmic stimuli. Most horses become habituated quickly to the finger in the nose, and from there it's just a simple step to substitute the tube for the finger. How long

11

it takes depends on the horse's disposition, and how badly spoiled he is. When the stomach tube hits the back of the throat, a new stimulus is added; he gags, and that often will frighten him. But the reassurance of the other stimuli helps him quickly adjust to the new sensations as the tube passes into his stomach.

The next point I'd like to discuss in understanding the horse's mind concerns his ability to choose between the "lesser of two evils." When a horse is offered a choice between a frightening, non-painful stimulus, and a frightening painful stimulus, he will choose the former, unless he has become so frightened of something in his past that he would rather suffer pain than face that particular non-painful but frightening stimulus.

Let's say we wish a horse to cross a stream, and he's never crossed a stream before. In order to persuade him to cross, the rider uses the whip or spur, which are frightening, painful stimuli. If properly used, the horse will learn that he can escape the unpleasant stimulus by moving toward the water.

The skilled trainer will use the whip or spur to elicit forward movement. Once that response is constant, the horse is asked to step forward toward the thing he fears (in this case, the water). One step is all the rider asks for, and that is immediately rewarded by relaxing the pressure, and by rewarding words and petting. The slightest response toward the water should be rewarded, and the horse must not be rushed. If the training is done correctly, the horse will soon realize that security lies *toward* the water.

The unskilled rider will continue to apply whip or spur even when the horse approaches the water. When this happens, the horse figures that he can't escape the painful stimulus whether he moves toward the water or not, so why go into it? He thinks, "I *thought* that might hurt me, and sure enough, when I go near it I get hurt!" Thus the horse acquires an adverse reaction to water forevermore.

The same technique is used to teach a horse to load into a trailer, or enter a frightening dark stall, or go into a confining treatment stocks, or for accepting any other non-painful stimulus that frightens him. Again, the only time this method will fail is if the horse had his fears reinforced when he previously encountered that experience. Then the horse might prefer the painful stimulus, but that's a spoiled horse, and we're not talking about that.

Obviously, it is preferable to get the horse used to things like trailers and streams and anything else that is potentially frightening, long before he is broke to ride. That's a great help, but inevitably the green horse is going to experience sights and sounds that frighten him and that he must learn to tolerate.

The lesser-of-two-evils approach can be used in many ways. Suppose, for example, our problem is a horse that is hard to catch. When approached, he persistently turns his back and runs away, and can be caught only with a bucket of grain. Such behavior is often initially caused by fear, and later the horse learns that he can outrun man. Eventually he will refuse to be caught because he has learned an evasive behavior pattern, even though he is no longer afraid.

A good way to correct this bad habit is to confine the horse in a relatively small pen, perhaps 30 to 50 feet in diameter. Approach the horse with a light whip or a length of rope in hand. As soon as the horse starts to move away, go after him in a threatening manner. Frighten him and keep him in constant motion around the pen (be sure the fence is high enough and strong enough so that he can't escape). Watch his head carefully. Sooner or later he will, in desperation, stop looking for an escape route *outside of the pen*, and will glance at you.

The moment he does so, immediately lower the threatening whip, step backwards away *from the horse, and assume a quiet, passive stance.*

If your reactions are swift enough, the horse will quickly realize (usually after the third time), that safety lies *toward* you and not *away* from you. He will soon face you and may even take a step toward you. You can encourage this by taking a step *away* from him.

Reward any movement toward you, however slight, with soothing words and encouragement. If he panics and starts to run, resume your aggressive posture and go after him again, but be sure to *in-*

stantly reward his slightest movement toward you (even if it's just a glance) by stepping backward and assuming a passive and non-threatening posture. Eventually you will be able to scratch his nose, pet him, and finally, halter him.

After the halter is on, *then* reward him with a snack. Then turn him loose, give him a few minutes to digest the experience, and then repeat the whole performance. In a few days your horse will be easy to catch, and may even come up to you when you approach with the halter.

As a practicing vet, I have had to cope with many head-shy horses, and this is a problem when I want to examine a mouth, pass a stomach tube up a nostril, or do dentistry. Most head-shy horses get that way as youngsters, when they are frightened by someone's crude attempts to handle, halter, bridle, or somehow restrain their heads. As soon as a colt learns that he can escape by throwing his head in the air, the behavior pattern becomes fixed and reinforced. If frustrated handlers then become angry and use brute force to accomplish their ends, the horse's original fears become intensified and reinforced.

This is how I re-educate such a horse. I apply a lip chain, or in some cases a war bridle, to the horse. There are many ways of rigging war bridles, but all of them cause severe discomfort when tension is applied to the lead rope, as does the lip chain, and for this reason a person must exercise exceptionally good judgment when using them.

I stand close to the horse quietly, talk to him and pet him to reduce his fear. Gradually, I let my hand approach his mouth; perhaps I want to examine his teeth. He immediately throws up his head to escape the hand, and the war bridle or lip chain causes immediate pain. I didn't hurt him; he hurt himself by throwing up his head. This frightens him, and when he calms down, I try again. Depending on the horse's intelligence and his disposition, and how badly spoiled he is, he soon learns to associate the pain of the bridle with the throwing of his head, not with my approaching hand.

Most horses will learn with three attempts. Some cases, of course, are much more difficult. Even though the horse has long had the habit of throwing his head, putting it out of reach, he will soon accept the lesser of two evils, the least frightening alternative. Once he accepts my hand, I reinforce the lesson by not hurting with my hand; in fact, I pet him and praise him. Again, the trainer must be consistent, must control his temper, must comprehend the horse's mind and reactions. As a man once said, "In order to teach a horse anything, you must first be smarter than the horse."

But it is not enough to be smarter than the horse if you don't establish dominance over him.

In the wild, horses exist in bands or herds, and like all animals living in such colonies, the leadership is assumed by a strongly dominant animal. Dominance does not simply mean that the leader can outfight and defeat any other horse in the herd. There is more to it than simple fighting strength, aggressiveness, and fighting skill. Dominance also involves an indefinable quality of character, a leadership factor to which the rest of the herd submits.

Some people are offended by the concept of *dominating* the horse. Please understand, domination does *not* imply the use of force, or cruelty, or physical violence. Submissiveness is a state of mind, and the horse *must* be submissive to be useful to the person using the horse.

To establish who dominates, it is ordinarily assumed that the human will dominate the animal, but such isn't always the case. It isn't unusual, for example, for a family dog to dominate a family, except for one individual he recognizes as master. In some cases, the animal may dominate the entire family. Many horse owners don't understand that it's necessary to dominate the horse if he is to be useful. Such owners, especially women and girls, think their horses will work for them for love alone. This isn't so. Since many horses are highly submissive, the owner is under the impression that the horse performs because of affection.

An owner with a low dominance factor will dominate a horse if the horse has an even lower dominance factor. This matter of dominance and submissiveness is important to understand, because its existence is what makes the horse as a

> **Many horse owners don't understand that it's necessary to dominate the horse if he is to be useful.**

13

species useful to us, and also explains why some horses are difficult or impossible to break.

It's an integral part of the horse's nature to accept dominance; except for the rare, superdominant individual, horses *want* to be dominated. They are willing to let the leader of the band make the decisions, and will follow along blindly. The submissive horse—and remember again this has nothing to do with brains or brawn—can be a great athlete and highly intelligent. Such a horse is easy to train. Horsemen often speak of kind horses, honest horses, willing horses, gentle horses. These horses are usually submissive.

The dominant horse is harder to break in training. The trainer must establish dominance over the horse before the horse will be responsive. If the trainer is submissive, and the horse is dominant, the trainer is in trouble. Such a horse does what he wants to do. If he doesn't want to do something, he becomes difficult. Strongly dominant horsemen are naturals, and most horses respond to them well. Less dominant horsemen have more problems relating to dominant horses. Some get along by assuming an aura of dominance, but few people are that good at acting, and most horses are far too intelligent to be fooled.

Superdominant horses make outlaws. They're tough-minded mounts that challenge man's right to make them do anything. Submissive horses, like submissive people, are easy-going and pleasant to get along with. Highly dominant people make great leaders, but they may be difficult to work with. I've heard that teachers rarely like highly dominant children; the horse and trainer relationship is duplicated in kindergarten. Strongly dominant horses, however, "taught" by skilled and domineering trainers, make superb working horses.

I want to repeat again: Don't confuse dominance with cruelty or physical aggressiveness. As an analogy, many strongly dominant humans aren't physically aggressive. These may include great statesmen, teachers, spiritual leaders, clergymen, and entertainers. Of course, if dominance is combined with aggressiveness, it creates in either the horse or the human an ominous individual. Adolph Hitler was such a personality, and I once knew a horse just like him.

Some people have a personality that horses respond to with almost automatic submissiveness. These people may or may not display dominance in their relationships with other people, or even with other animals. But they are naturally dominant with horses. They're exceptional horsemen who "just have a way with horses," and they make excellent trainers and handlers. Although few people are born with this natural ability, every horseman can be taught how to dominate most horses. I don't believe that the techniques can be fully explained in writing alone. They must also be demonstrated and practiced. However, I will mention a few general principles.

I have repeatedly pointed out that the horse's principal means of survival, his most natural instinct, is instantaneous flight—the "fearful flight" reaction. And whenever the ability of the horse to flee is taken from him, it has a profound effect on his determination.

Old-time horse breakers subdued an outlaw horse by tying him down on soft ground, and establishing dominance over the animal by crawling all over him, slapping, rubbing, sacking him out, all while the horse was helplessly restrained. When released, the formerly intractable horse usually exhibited complete submissiveness to the handler. One word of caution—such methods are only for the real expert. No ordinary horseman should ever attempt such a dangerous technique. I mentioned it only to further explain the psychological effects involved. Less drastic means of depriving a horse of his ability to flee can be used by any horseman to establish dominance. Common examples are a halter and lead chain, hobbles, and the use of a longe line and cavesson.

I sometimes use an interesting technique on horses that I can't handle because they lack submissiveness, or are so strongly dominant that they actually threaten me. I quietly tie up one foreleg with a strong, specially constructed one-leg hobble. Years ago, a Randy Steffen "Handy Hint" in *Western Horseman* showed such a hobble. I made one up from that, and it worked far better than

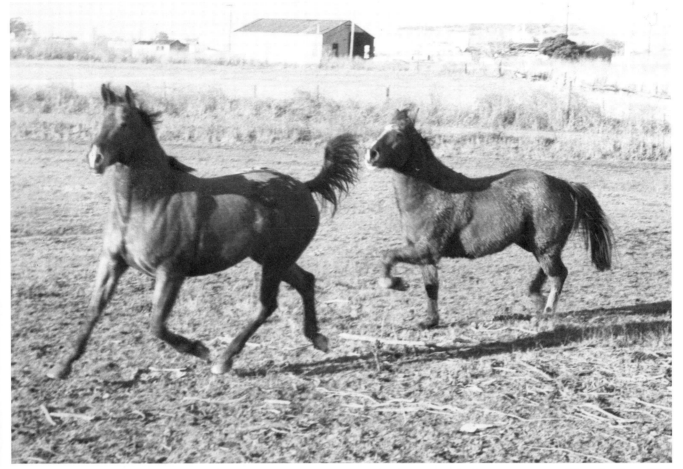

Photo by Caron Kirk

what I had used previously. You can use a soft cotton rope for a one-leg hobble, or you can also use an English stirrup leather.

This should always be done in a well-fenced enclosure on soft ground, because some horses will drop to one knee when attempting to regain the use of the immobilized leg. Once in a great while, a horse will lie down in his frustration. In extremely rare cases, a horse might throw himself while fighting the hobble. Most horses will struggle violently to get the leg free, and perhaps hop around the corral. Before long they stop struggling, and stand dejectedly. Fatigue sets in after a few minutes, and the horse starts to shake and sweat. At this point, I quietly approach him, hold him by the halter and lead rope with one hand, and release the hobble with my free hand. What relief! I allow the horse to take a step or two forward, then I reapply the hobble and walk away.

The horse has now learned that I have powers he can't comprehend. I can immobilize one leg and I can restore its function. After a few more minutes, I

return to the horse. He's glad to see me, and I reward him by releasing the hobble and walking him around. In most cases the formerly aggressive and unruly horse will lower his head against my chest in a submissive attitude. The fire has left his eyes. He's now submissive and will accept me as his dominating leader. If he doesn't, I simply repeat the hobbling lesson until the horse is convinced that I have God-like powers. If necessary, I do it on both forelegs. All of this is done without shouting, fussing, or threatening, or losing my temper. Only the most severe type of outlaw requires more drastic subduing techniques.

Most horses, in fact, never require the use of the one-leg hobble. They are usually submissive enough that if they are properly halter-broke, the use of the halter alone renders them psychologically impotent and submissive to the skilled handler. Let me give a very common example. Many mares, immediately after foaling, will exhibit aggressiveness toward any approaching human. In the majority of cases, if the mare is once caught and haltered, her

15

attitude immediately changes toward the person handling her, and while she still shows great concern for her foal, she will no longer demonstrate aggressiveness.

Perhaps something should be said about what constitutes a properly halter-broke horse. The beginning of all training, whether for a colt or an older horse, starts with correct halter breaking. And a properly halter-broke horse won't pull back or fight the halter; he will lead wherever the halter takes him, whether he's being led from another horse, from a vehicle, tied to the back of a wagon, or led by a man or child on foot. If properly halter-broke, he submits to that alone, and it totally alters his attitude toward everything because he has a feeling of helplessness and dependency on the human that he doesn't have when he's loose.

Horsemen have seen this attitude in horses in a corral or pasture, running and defying the human until they're caught. Then they seem to say, "Okay, you've got me; the rules of the game are now that I have to be a good boy and do whatever you want." This is submissiveness. And this is what the halter and these other devices are capable of doing.

Many training techniques utilize this psychological effect on the horse. Training horses on the longe line or driving them on long lines, aside from teaching response to the various signals, also renders them submissive to their trainer because their natural ability to flee danger has been removed.

In the old bronc-busting days of the early West, not much emphasis was given to avoid frightening a horse, and in fact, some of the breaking techniques made the horse permanently fearful of man, and hence permanently untrustworthy. A heavy emphasis was placed on establishing dominance over the horse and making the horse submissive to man, and the principal techniques used were to remove the horse's ability to flee. Consequently, the horse was first taught to respect a lariat rope; and when caught and snubbed to the snubbing post, he learned that he could not escape. A horse was hobbled prior to being saddled and ridden, and sometimes blindfolded. All of these things interfered with his ability to escape enemies.

I have used the term hobble not only to indicate the tying together of legs, but also the tying up of a leg. In early bronc-breaking days, cowboys would frequently tie up, or "scotch" up, a hind leg, or tie up a front leg. The principle is the same, and many horsemen still use these methods. A lot of people think this is to prevent the horse from kicking, but that's not the whole story. It psychologically dominates the horse; it renders impotent his instinct to flee.

Good horse trainers establish, at an early stage of schooling, two means of control over the horse. These are lateral flexion of the head, and the ability to control the hind end by displacing it laterally. For those not familiar with these two techniques. I will briefly explain.

Lateral flexion of the head is obtained, using halter, hackamore, or bridle, by pulling the horse's head to one side or the other until resistance ceases and the horse will softly yield his head all the way around to either side. This is obtained a little at a time, rewarding any relaxation with an immediate release from pressure. Once the horse consistently and lightly yields the head to either side, the goal of lateral flexion is obtained.

Similarly, the horse should respond to flank pressure (via the heel or the leg), by moving his hind end laterally. This can be taught from the ground, or from the saddle, again asking for only a step at first, and immediately rewarding by releasing the pressure. When the horse lightly and consistently moves his hind end laterally, the goal is obtained. Of course, this takes patience and many lessons.

What is the purpose of all this? The trainer will explain that these steps establish *control* over the horse. Why? Because a horse *cannot resort to flight in a straight line*, his natural response to fear, once these two means of control are well established.

The horse that flexes laterally will circle when he attempts to move out. The horse whose hind end can be immediately displaced to the side with leg pressure cannot run off, cannot buck, and cannot rear.

Forward motion in a four-legged animal is achieved by propulsion. The hind end powers forward movement. If the

16

Photo by Jean Latimer

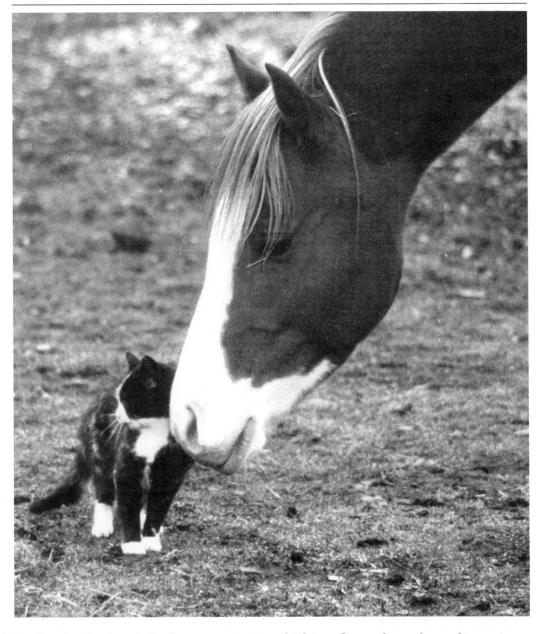

hind end is displaced, the horse, again, is deprived of his primary survival mechanism—flight.

Thus, absolute control of the head and the hindquarters, early in training, not only enables us to control the *direction* of travel, but it again makes the horse submissive in attitude by removing his primary survival technique. This is why the old-time hackamore man *doubled* his colt. It rendered the animal submissive.

Now a word about the aggressive horse. When a horse can't escape from danger, when he is startled and feels he must protect himself because he doesn't have time to run away, or because he knows that he is tied or confined to an area too small to permit escape, he might defend himself by striking, biting, or

kicking. Once a horse learns he can intimidate humans by such behavior, once he learns his own strength, once he learns that humans can be fearful and weak, then the behavior is reinforced, and we have the origins of a serious problem—the aggressive horse. Aggression toward humans can be prevented by immediately and severely punishing the horse, but the timing must be appropriate. The experienced horseman is always on guard against such behavior from a strange horse.

The occasional colt that shows a tendency to present his hind end to a human, and kick or threaten to kick, must be discouraged by immediately and severely whacking him across the hind end with a rope or a whip. Only one blow should be inflicted unless it fails to turn the threatening kicker aside. The colt must learn to associate his antisocial behavior with almost simultaneous punishment. If one must run to the barn for a whip, the punishment is useless.

For punishment to be effective, the horse must assume that he is punishing himself. He thinks, "Every time I cock a hind leg at that guy, my hind end gets stung." Or he might think, "Every time I charge somebody with teeth bared, my nose gets stung." As always, the horse will accept the lesser of two evils. It is best to deliver the punishment with no word or reprimand. Let the horse think he's hurting himself. This is why I say I rarely punish a horse: I allow the horse to punish himself.

I have cured a number of cow-kicking horses by standing at the shoulder, out of reach, and almost simultaneously as the horse kicked forward at me, delivered a hard kick at the belly with the side of my boot (never the toe). I make no sound or comment as I do so. The horse seems to think he's kicked his own belly. After a couple of kicks, he usually tries a third, less-enthusiastic, part-way kick. That too results in an immediate, uncomfortable blow. Then he might tentatively elevate the leg part way as if he's thinking about cow-kicking. These attempts always result in injuring his own belly. Most horses quickly decide to give it up at this point. The psychological principles involved are the same—reward and punishment. In some cases, the reward is simply to stop the punishment.

Finally, I'm going to mention a rather audacious technique of getting along with horses, which in all sincerity, is probably beyond the capabilities of all but a few readers. When someone constantly works with horses and observes them closely, he becomes aware of the methods by which horses communicate with one another. These include a wide variety of vocalized sounds, postural attitudes, and tactile stimuli such as nibbling or bumping with the nose. I use such "horse talk" to help me get along with horses. It's possible to reassure, to intimidate, to threaten, and to dominate horses with mimicry if one cares to learn the techniques—all it takes is thousands of hours with thousands of horses.

Learning to nicker a friendly greeting to a horse, to use your fingers to "nibble" a horse's neck, to squeal and kick like a stallion might enhance your ability to communicate with horses. Don't be surprised, however, if your neighbors begin to regard you with a suspicious eye.

The illustration on page 20 shows my one-leg hobble, which is made of double-stitched latigo leather with a roller buckle for quick release. It will work on any size horse, but sometimes will not stay in position on a heavily muscled Quarter Horse.

To apply the hobble, I put a loop in the strap, pick up the foot, slip the loop around the pastern, and buckle the strap around the forearm. The horse does not realize he is being hobbled. I continue holding the foot for a few seconds, talking to the horse and petting him; then I ease away. Some horses stand quietly; some hop around on three legs for a few minutes; and a few have charged me. If I suspect that might happen, I put an extra-long lead rope on the horse so I can whack him on the nose when he charges and make him back off. If the horse is in a small, safe enclosure, I sometimes turn him loose for ten minutes. Then I catch him and release the hobble for a few minutes before reapplying it.

Some horses are so spoiled, or afraid of a veterinarian, that it can be difficult to get near them to put the hobble on. With such a horse, I've found he is less likely to run backwards if I approach him in a stooped-over position. Evidently that makes me seem less threatening to him. When I get next to him, I can usually pick his foot up; then he will relax a little because he thinks maybe I'm a horseshoer, and I can go ahead and apply the hobble.

Examine Your Horse

Just as every good mother learns to evaluate her child's health by the youngster's attitude, appetite, skin tone, and by feeling the forehead for signs of fever, so must the horse owner learn to evaluate the horse's health. There are certain signs one can look for that quickly signal that a horse isn't well, but in order to recognize these signs, one must first be familiar with the normals. If we are not thoroughly familiar with normal functions, and the normal appearance of the horse, we cannot identify the abnormal when it is presented. In this discussion, I will try to help the reader become familiar with the normal.

APPETITE: Watch several horses at feeding time. Note the alacrity with which they start to eat. Do horses keep on eating until they are full? Or, do they munch a while, and then wander away, to return again later?

Any time a horse refuses to eat at feeding time, something is wrong. Take the horse's temperature. Is there a fever? If the temperature is normal, observe the horse for signs of colic. Laying down, rolling, cramping, stretching as if to urinate, and lifting the upper lip are all signs of possible colic. If colic is present, remove all food and call a veterinarian.

TEMPERATURE: Buy a rectal thermometer. Take the temperature of a half-dozen normal, healthy horses. Insert the thermometer two-thirds its length. Leave it in for three minutes. Remove it, wipe it off, and read it. Write the temperatures down. Add them up, and find the average. You now know the average rectal temperature of the horse, and have observed the normal variations that can occur.

PULSE: Most easily taken by most people by putting the ear (or a stethoscope) to the left rib cage, just behind and above the point of the elbow. Take the pulse of a half-dozen quiet, relaxed horses. What is the average pulse rate? Slow, isn't it? About a third the rate of your own.

ABDOMINAL SOUNDS: While you're listening to the chest, move back to the belly. Listen to the sounds for a full minute, on each side of the abdomen of a half-dozen horses. Remember what a normal belly sounds like. In cases of colic, those sounds are usually either greatly increased, or greatly diminished; and they may change their character completely, to sound like a "tinkle." The more bellies you listen to, the more competent you will become to evaluate abnormal sounds.

MUCUS MEMBRANES: Look at the gum color and the mucus membranes of the eyes of a couple of dozen healthy horses. Many horse owners are completely unfamiliar with what normal membranes look like. Look at them, not on one horse, but on many horses. See the variation in horses of different colors? After studying the mucus membranes of many horses, you will be able to recognize such abnormalities as paleness, jaundice (yellowing), cyanosis (purpling), and injection or muddiness (darkening and dullness).

While you're looking at the gums, press your finger against the gum. See how it blanches? How long does it take for the pale spot to resume normal color? This is called *capillary refill time.* Do it again. Count the seconds. Now do it on ten more horses. You now know the normal CRT. In illness, the CRT is often decreased. In some diseases, it can be increased. The CRT is an important way of evaluating a horse's state of health.

SOUNDNESS OF GAIT: This is a good thing to study at a horse show. Watch several dozen horses trot. Don't look at the entire horse. Don't look at the rider. Just watch the head. It should, at the trot, bob up and down evenly with each stride. If there is a forelimb lameness, the head will go down on the sound limb. This is how we evaluate soundness. Don't look at the leg. Look at the head, and do it at a trot. Look at enough trotting horses, and you will soon be surprised to note how many of them are off in one front foot. I can't even enjoy the Rose Bowl Parade on TV because, by force of habit, I keep picking out lame horses as I watch. In fact, some of them are usually patients of mine. The same thing happens to me when I watch a western movie.

If a horse is lame in both forelimbs, then the gait will be choppy and short-strided, but rarely is a horse equally lame in both forelimbs. Usually, one leg is lamer than the other, and you'll still see the nose bob down when the less painful limb strikes the ground, putting more weight on it. Here's a rhyme to help you remember: "Down is sound."

It is more difficult to detect a hind limb lameness. You must watch the top of the hips. The horse's hip will go down when the sound limb hits the ground; you must stare at the hind end of many trotting horses to acquire skill at detecting hind limb lameness. Always concentrate on the trot. Many lamenesses that are apparent at the trot will not be obvious at a walk, or at the faster gaits.

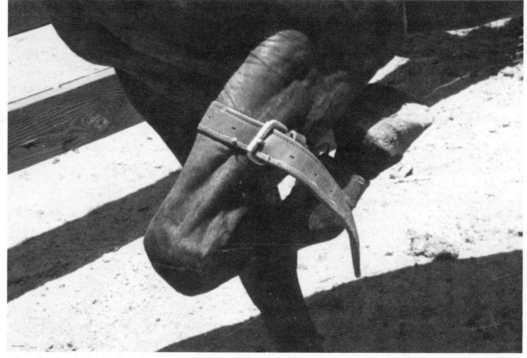

The one-leg hobble should go around the pastern and forearm. Use it with caution and do not leave it on longer than ten minutes at a time as a general rule.

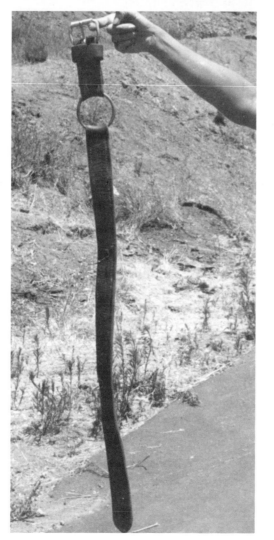

By familiarizing ourselves with the normal horse, the abnormal becomes apparent to us when we see it.

Restraint

When we speak of restraint in horsemanship, we refer to the techniques and tools used to control horses, to distract them, to immobilize them, to prevent them from injuring themselves or others, and to compel them to do our bidding.

Horses are much stronger physically than we are, but man's intelligence has led to the development of various devices by which we control the horse. We are all familiar with most of these; they include halters, hackamores, bits, spurs, and so on. But there are many more restraining devices less familiar to the casual horseman, which are used by professional horsemen to restrain the horse for purposes of breaking, treatment, and shoeing. A professional horseman is one who makes his living working with horses, and such a person, whether it be a farrier, a veterinarian, a horse-breaker, trainer, or cowboy, must be an expert in restraint. The professional knows that in order to work on some horses special restraint techniques are needed.

My experience as an equine practitioner has taught me that the majority of amateur horsemen do *not* understand the purpose, need, or methods of restraint. The amateur horseman loves horses, and when he sees a professional apply restraint, he interprets it as being "cruel." He regards his horse as gentle, and when he sees the professional use a chain shank or some other means of restraint, he considers it unnecessary.

Adult humans allow the doctor to poke and examine them, and the dentist to perform painful procedures. But what about a two-year-old child? He might kick and fight and scream. In fact he might act that way when he gets his first haircut because he is frightened and unfamiliar with what is happening. Even if it doesn't hurt, he *thinks* it will. Well, that's exactly how a colt feels the first time he is shod, or when the veterinarian worms him. We can overpower the child and *force* him to stay in the barber's chair. But that thousand-pound colt may require a twitch or other restraining device if he hasn't been previously trained to tolerate the procedure in question.

Another statement one often hears about a veterinarian or shoer is that "he is afraid of horses." This idea originates when the amateur observes the professional horseman working around a horse with habitual caution, or using a restraining device. Common sense should tell the owner in question that a man doesn't choose to spend his life working with horses if he fears them. A safer and more profitable living can be made elsewhere.

Rather than criticizing the shoer or veterinarian, the amateur should realize that this person handles thousands of horses every year, and should try to learn *how* and *why* he or she handles horses that way.

The horse's great value to man lies in his great strength, agility, and speed. But these very attributes that make the horse so useful can also make him *dangerous*. Automobiles, airplanes, firearms, and boats can also be dangerous if handled carelessly by untrained and inexperienced people. When handled properly, observing the rules of safety, all of these things, and the horse as well, can provide us with great pleasure.

So let's decide to learn how to handle horses correctly, both in the saddle and on the ground.

I was fortunate in that many of the first horses I worked with were range broncs. They were unpredictable and sometimes dangerous, and caution and good safety habits were deeply instilled in me. In later years, working at the racetrack, breaking colts, and rodeoing, I learned more about handling horses with care and respect. Finally, as a veterinarian, I acquired the greatest experience possible, because a veterinarian must handle horses that are sick, hurt, and frightened and often his treatments are uncomfortable for the horse. Horseshoers have similar problems. The veterinarian or horseshoer who isn't an expert at restraining a horse is soon injured.

The most potentially dangerous horse is the gentle horse. You see, only an expert will try to handle a vicious stud or a green bronc, and he approaches such a horse with due respect. But the gentle horse is trusted by his owner. He grows careless. He forgets the rules, or possibly doesn't know them. When that horse is exposed to a frightening stimulus that he is unfamiliar with, he will respond by either running away from it, or by attacking it with a kick or strike. This is how amateur horsemen get hurt, and this is why a professional horseman moves carefully, or uses restraint when indicated. The amateur may interpret this as fear.

Most veterinarians can tell you that when a horse they are treating blows up, they are rarely injured, but the inattentive owner frequently is hurt. That's because we expect trouble, and are prepared for it, whereas the owner may not be. We often apply a hobble, or sideline a horse, to protect the *owner* who is assisting us, and we have to constantly remind such people to stay alert, stand to the side, and keep out of the line of fire.

Now that we understand the reason for restraint, let's consider a few of the methods so that you can assist your veterinarian or horseshoer, or so that you can treat your horse yourself, when necessary.

The horse requiring medical attention should always be wearing a halter equipped with a lead rope. A bridle or a rope around the neck, even with a halfhitch around the nose, is inferior to a well-fitting halter. Don't *ever* treat a horse that is loose. *Always* have the head under control. It is best not to tie the head. It should be held. A hurt or frightened horse tied by the head may pull back and injure himself. Never stand directly in front of the patient. *Always* stand at the side, preferably at the shoulder, and stay *close* to the horse. When you're at the shoulder and have the head under control with a halter, you are very unlikely to be struck or kicked. Remember this safety position.

For many minor procedures the horse can be distracted and calmed by the voice. But speak soothingly. Shouting "Ho! Ho! Boy! Ho!" won't calm anybody. Jiggling the lead rope often helps to distract a horse, as does the touch of a firm hand on the shoulder or on the neck in front of the withers.

The single most useful restraint device used on horses is the twitch. A chain twitch is less severe (when handled properly) than a rope twitch because the rope can twist up deceptively tight, whereas with the chain, one can *feel* the degree of tension. Handling a twitch properly is an art and I won't attempt to explain it in writing. Buy a twitch (be sure it has a long handle) or make one, and then have a professional demonstrate its use to you. Remember that *most* horses will become immobilized when twitched, but not *all* of them. Some horses react adversely to a twitch. Usually such horses may be controlled by "earing them down." However, there are horses on which neither method works. In fact, there are horses so head-shy that one cannot get hold of either the lip or ear. Proper twitching and earing *will not* make a horse head-shy. Always release slowly, and then gently massage the ear or lip. This will facilitate the procedure the next time it is required.

Although the twitch is an indispensable and legitimate means of restraint, it is often misused. Frequently a horse will allow a procedure to be done if we just go at it slowly and back off a bit when the horse shows fear. Our retreating for a moment reassures the horse and a second or third attempt is often successful when the first attempt caused the horse to panic or evade us due to fear.

The secret to working with horses is to dominate them without *eliciting a fearful reaction which usually precipitates a* *flight response. However, when restraint is necessary, it should be applied properly, and without anger or haste, which will further alarm the horse.*

The illustrations accompanying this discussion demonstrate a few of the simple restraint methods that may be used by the average horse owner, *when* and *if* needed. Many more elaborate methods such as war bridles, etc., are known to every professional. Lastly, we are fortunate to live in an age of tranquilizing drugs, anesthetics, and immobilizing drugs, and while these have become indispensable to the practitioner, they by no means eliminate the need for simple physical restraint. Horses are animals, and as long as men cause them discomfort or fear with the hypodermic needle or examiner's hand, certain horses will require a twitch or an ear hold. The experienced horseman sizes the horse up quickly and accurately. Don't question his choice of restraint. If he didn't know his business he'd soon be maimed or killed, or in some other line of work.

Tranquilizing Horses

I will never forget the first horse I tranquilized. Many years ago I was called to treat a huge Thoroughbred that was notoriously high-strung and a very difficult patient. Something had spooked him in his stall, and he had jumped high enough to scalp himself on a ceiling beam. I had to stand on a stump to examine the wound, and he was so jumpy that I could not touch him.

In my bag I had a vial of tranquilizer for human use, which was then being experimentally tried in horses. Apprehensively, I injected the drug intravenously. Within ten minutes I was amazed and pleased to find him completely docile, head hanging low, enabling me to repair the wound very easily. I realized then that tranquilizing drugs would soon revolutionize equine medicine, and that these drugs would have many uses—and misuses—in the years to come.

Today, every horseman knows about tranquilizers, and most horsemen have had experience with these drugs. But many misconceptions exist about them.

Of the many tranquilizers available, I have found a few that are dependable in the horse. The first and oldest of these is

Promazine hydrochloride. It is marketed in the United States under the trade names of *Promazine* and *Sparine.* Promazine hydrochloride is available as an injectable solution for intramuscular or intravenous use, and also in granular or pelleted form for oral use.

Acepromazine maleate is a reliable tranquilizer. It requires a very small injection to produce a maximum of sedation with a minimum of accompanying grogginess.

Rompun (trade name for xylazine) is another excellent tranquilizer.

There are other tranquilizers used in horses. Some of these are legal and labelled for equine use, and others are being used illegally. A number of other experimental tranquilizers are in the mill. Some of these may soon be available.

Tranquilizers are drugs with several effects on the body. They act on the brain to relieve excitability, nervousness, anxiety, and fear. They also relieve nausea and motion sickness, and cause general relaxation. Please understand that tranquilizers allay fear. *You cannot train a horse with a tranquilizer.* If, for example, a horse has never been loaded in a trailer, and is afraid to load, a tranquilizer may reduce his anxiety, but it cannot teach him to load. What I am trying to say is that tranquilizers are not substitutes for training. Too many people expect them to be.

Tranquilizers are very useful to veterinarians. We use them to calm the frightened patient, and as pre- and post-operative medication. They are useful drugs to horsemen for transporting high-strung stock, especially young, green horses. Tranquilizers may simplify weaning and other procedures that cause agitation in some horses.

Unfortunately, and inevitably, tranquilizers are being used by some horsemen in ways that are questionable and sometimes downright immoral. For example, an unscrupulous horse trader can pass off a horse with poor temperament on an unsuspecting buyer by tranquilizing the horse prior to the sale. Experienced persons can usually detect a horse under the influence of drugs, but many buyers lack this experience.

Tranquilizing show horses is a questionable procedure in many cases. It is true that many good-dispositioned young horses get a little excited at a show, especially if they haven't been to many, and such behavior is understandable. In my personal opinion, there isn't a great deal of harm done to the breed by taking the edge off such a colt with a little tranquilizer; however, horse show rules do not allow the tranquilizing of any horses.

The vile-tempered or excessively high-strung broodmare or stallion also represent a matter of ethics. It would be possible, by tranquilizing such individuals, to conceal their defective behavior, and establish them as halter class winners. Since disposition faults are often inheritable, you can see that the use of tranquilizers could, in time, be detrimental to the temperament of the entire breed.

Most major breed associations, as well as the American Horse Shows Association, have strict rules regarding any drug use. If you show, familiarize yourself with the drug rules of the particular association sanctioning each show. Blood tests are available to detect tranquilizers in questionable situations.

Tranquilizers, being psychological drugs, are variable in their effect on different individuals. The dosage may vary from one horse to another. Or, one tranquilizer might be more effective than another in a given horse. Occasionally, a tranquilizer will have an adverse effect on certain horses. Instead of becoming tranquil, such horses might become very excited, or even aggressive. These variations in the effects of tranquilizers are rare, but they do occur—not only in horses, but in other animals, and in humans as well.

The tranquilizers I have mentioned very rarely cause these undesirable reactions. There are many other tranquilizers on the market, and while they work very well in other species, they are not safe to use in horses. These other tranquilizers might work well in the horse, but they are much too prone to cause violent reactions. Improperly tranquilized horses have been known to go berserk, or to collapse. Therefore, follow your veterinarian's advice before you attempt to tranquilize a horse.

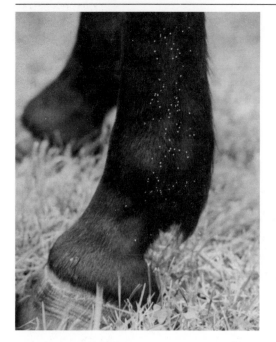

Those little yellow specks on your horse's legs are bot eggs. They can be scraped off with a sharp knife or a razor blade.

Deworming

Worming is vitally important. Next to proper nutrition, control of internal parasites is the most important facet of horse husbandry. Yet some horse owners ignore parasite control completely, or delude themselves into thinking they are taking care of the problem by giving the horse a dose of worm medicine once a year or so.

Nearly all horses have worms. These worms rob the horse of vitality, and increase the owner's feed bill. They damage the arteries, causing horses to die before their time. They cause colics and obstructions in the digestive tract. They interfere with the growth and development of young horses, and cause lung damage. They are involved in the production of summer sores and other skin disease.

Horsemen tend to ignore these facts because they can't see the worms. Only when the worms are seen in the manure do some horse owners take action. Yet, a horse may be heavily parasitized without the owner knowing about it. Many owners erroneously think that as long as a horse is fat, there is no need to worm him. The fact is that horses, like wild animals and primitive humans, are almost universally parasitized. Since worm eggs and larvae are passed in the manure, horses confined to paddocks, corrals, or stalls are subject to constant reinfestation.

Keeping these parasites under control is a perpetual battle, and even with the finest drugs and most conscientious program, it is a difficult job to do well. Remember that nature has provided the parasite with a unique mode of existence. He depends upon his host for survival. He must rob his host in order to live, but he defeats his own purpose if his host dies. For this reason, most horses go through life supporting internal parasites and being robbed by them, while the owner ignores the problem simply because he cannot see it.

In the United States, horses are widely infested by several types of worms. Several other types occur less commonly.

Strongyles (bloodworms) are found in nearly all horses. They are quite small. The eggs are passed in the manure and cannot be seen without a microscope, as is the case with all the worms we will discuss. They severely damage the intestines and the blood vessels. The bloodworm is unquestionably the most serious and widespread parasite of the horse.

Ascarids (roundworms) are large white worms most common in young foals. They rob the foal of vitality, and the migrating larvae can cause lung damage, a cough, and nasal discharge.

Oxyuris (pinworms) are not very dangerous, but they do cause itching of the hind end, with subsequent tail rubbing.

Other worms found in horses include *Habronema (large stomach worms)*, the larvae of which produce summer sores, and *Trichostrongylus (small stomach worms)*, *Strongyloides*, and *tapeworms*.

There is one very common internal parasite of the horse that is not a worm at all, but the larvae of a fly. This is the *bot (Gastrophilus)*. This grub-like creature lives in the stomach. After eight or ten months it passes out of the horse and burrows into the soil, to emerge a month later as a fly. The female bot fly then lays her eggs on the hair of the horse where they appear as little yellow specks. (They can be scraped off with a razor blade or sharp knife.) They hatch tiny larvae that enter the mouth of the horse and burrow into the gums. After another month they emerge and pass to the stomach where they attach, feed, and grow.

The varieties of internal parasites, their life cycles, and the susceptibilities to various drugs vary tremendously from one area to another. Nobody understands the problem more fully than your local equine practitioner. He or she knows what month of the year to attack the bots in your area to get a maximum kill. He'll tell you which of the three varieties of bots to look for, and how to remove the eggs. He knows what formula works on the worms occurring in your community, and which formulas they have become immune to. You see, these worms can develop resistance to medication, just as flies grow resistant to insecticides.

The veterinarian, by running microscopic fecal examinations, is able to evaluate the effects of various medications. He knows which ones work best, can determine the incidence of parasitism on each site, and work out a control program for the individual owner for saddle horses, broodmares, or young stock as the case may be. The medication he prescribes might be liquids to be administered through a stomach tube, boluses (tablets) to be given by mouth, or pastes or powders to mix with the feed.

Remember that there is no single product yet on the market in edible powder form that is effective against all the common parasites of the horse. Also remember that all of these drugs can produce toxic reactions, especially if used incorrectly.

For the old-timers, let's get one thing straight: Tobacco and garlic are not effective vermifuges. If they were, then pharmaceutical companies and the U.S. government wouldn't be spending fortunes developing and testing new drugs for deworming horses.

There are a number of general points that must be remembered in establishing a parasite control program for horses:

1/ Horses must be wormed at regular intervals, several times a year, to keep them free of parasites. Keeping them free of parasites is very important to prevent damage to internal organs caused by the migration of parasitic larvae, to prevent colic, and to prevent shortening the horse's life.

2/ The specific schedule and the best drugs to use vary widely with the climate and the environment. The best person to consult for an effective program, therefore, is a veterinarian experi-enced in equine medicine who practices in your area.

3/ The dosages of vermifuges (worm-killing drugs) are weight-related. If a mistake is made when the horse's weight is estimated, or when the dose is calculated, the horse may be underdosed or overdosed. Underdosing will result in a failure to kill the worms. More important, underdosing creates resistance by the parasites to the medications used. It speeds their ability to become immune to the drugs. Overdosing, in moderate amounts, is safe with some drugs, but is dangerous with other drugs. Remember, ask your veterinarian to recommend a program.

4/ Paste wormers can be a useful part of your worm control program. Remember to:

A) Calculate the dose *accurately.* Paste wormers usually come in syringes in doses for 1,000-pound or 1,200-pound horses. Many of our modern saddle horses weigh more than 1,200 pounds. Big Thoroughbreds, Quarter Horses, and Warmbloods often weigh 1,400 pounds and some weigh considerably more.

B) Be sure there is no feed in the horse's mouth before you give a paste. The presence of feed will make it easy for the horse to spit out some of the paste, and there is no way for anyone to calculate how much of the dose the horse has lost.

5/ *Rotate wormers!* Nearly all parasitologists and veterinary experts recommend rotation to help prevent parasite resistance. And, ask local veterinarians which drugs are working and which are no longer working. If they have not recently tested the drugs to find out, you can do this yourself by having a microscopic fecal examination done on a sample of manure ten to fifteen days after the horse was wormed. There should be *no* worm eggs in the sample if the drug used was effective.

Remember that the companies that sell worming products are in business to make money, and they want to sell their product. So what the label says is not necessarily what is best for your horse. That's why we advise rotation of tested products and testing should be redone every two or three years to determine if resistance is developing.

The pharmaceutical industry has done an outstanding job during the last couple of decades in coming out with new and superior vermifuges. We can expect two things to continue in the years ahead:

A) By means of adaptation, parasites will continue to alter their life cycles and metabolisms to become resistant to most of the drugs currently being used.

B) Technology will continue to come up with new and different methods of parasite control.

External Parasites

Creatures that parasitize the horse externally include quite a variety of "bugs." Some of them are quite familiar; others are quite rare. But all of them are classified as parasites because they feed upon their host, thereby causing discomfort, loss of condition, and sometimes actual diseases.

Flies are certainly the most common equine parasite, and no stable is entirely free of them in the warmer months. The stable fly, horsefly, and housefly torment and bite horses. The screwworm fly lays its eggs on open wounds. Sand flies and gnats are a problem in some areas, as are face flies.

To combat the fly problem, it is necessary to have a manure disposal system as well as a fly control program. A wide variety of compounds are available for the latter purpose, and many of them are advertised in horse magazines. They include repellent products to apply directly on the horse, and insecticides to use in and around the stable. Fly baits and traps are also effective.

One word of caution: never use any of these products without first reading the label very carefully. Most fly control products are safe *if* used exactly as directed. Common sense must be used to ensure that no harm will come to children, pets, other animals, or the horses themselves. Read the label!

During fly season, protect wounds with appropriate fly repellent preparations that are safe to use on or near wounds, or by bandaging if necessary.

Mosquitoes not only feed upon horses, but also play an important role in transmitting sleeping sickness or encephalomyelitis. Therefore if mosquitoes are a problem, institute a control program that includes the use of repellents and insecticides, and treatment of ponds where mosquitoes breed.

Scabies, also known as scab or mange, is caused by tiny mites that burrow into the skin. They cause lesions that itch intensely, and the condition readily spreads to other parts of the body, or to other horses, especially by contaminated equipment. Itchy "rashes" should be examined by a veterinarian. He will differentiate scabies from other types of skin diseases. He does this by examining skin scrapings under the microscope, and looking for the tiny mites that cause the disease.

When scabies is diagnosed in a stable, a quarantine program should be started at once, and treatment given with appropriate medications.

Lice are tiny insects that spend their entire life cycle on the horse. They lay their eggs, known as "nits," on the hairs next to the skin. When these hatch, the lice feed upon the horse's skin.

There are two kinds of lice: biting and sucking. Sucking lice feed on the horse's blood, and in severe infestations can actually cause serious anemia. With biting lice, the skin is irritated and itchy, causing the horse to rub and bite the infested areas. As a result, large areas of skin become bald and raw. On close examination, nits and lice may both be seen.

Lice are most active in winter months and rarely cause any trouble in hot weather. Fortunately, they are easily destroyed by using insecticidal powders, dips, or sprays on the horse. Avoid contamination of mangers and feeding areas when treating the horse by doing this outside the stable or corral.

Ticks are a dangerous parasite because they carry a large number of diseases of humans and animals, including horses. Once premises are infested with ticks, they will become an increasingly severe problem. Therefore, prompt action should be taken to destroy ticks when they are first found on a horse. The owner will usually not see the "seed" or larval forms of the ticks, but rather the engorged tick attached to the skin.

When only occasional ticks are seen, the simplest way of handling them is to squirt them with a tick bomb (such as those made for dogs). Then they will die and fall off (in time). Applying lighted cigarettes or gasoline, or using other complex methods is unnecessary.

Where heavy infestations occur, spray or dip the horse in an insecticidal solution. Organic phosphates in proper dilution are effective. Again, many commercial preparations are available.

Ear ticks are especially troublesome in horses because they live deep down in the ear, causing great discomfort to the horse. Horses with ear ticks will shake their heads, rub their ears, and cock their heads from side to side. They become ear-shy and are hard to bridle.

These ticks are easily killed by instilling medication in the ear. It is necessary to restrain the horse with a twitch while doing this or he will not allow the medication to be put in the ear, or will immediately shake it out.

If the ears have been infested for a long time, there might be considerable debris and secondary infection present, necessitating veterinary attention.

Equine Dentistry

The teeth of a horse are different from those of most animals. They are extremely long, but only a small portion of the tooth protrudes into the mouth. A tooth might be likened to an iceberg: You can only see a small part of it.

The horse's teeth are constantly grinding coarse food; therefore they wear down. This is compensated for by continuous growth of the tooth. So the horse always has teeth to chew with, even though the chewing itself wears the tooth away. If a tooth is broken off, it will in time grow out to the point where it looks normal again. Due to this continuous growth, we can tell the age of a horse with reasonable accuracy, because the shape, angle, and markings of the tooth change as it grows.

Horses have "baby" teeth, also known as deciduous or milk teeth, as humans do. These are replaced by "adult" or permanent teeth. By five years of age, all of the permanent teeth are in, and the horse is said to have a "full mouth."

In the front of his mouth, the mature horse has six incisor teeth on top and six on the bottom. They are known as the first, second, and third (or central, middle, and corner) incisors. The purpose of

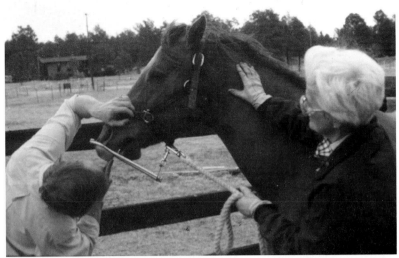

Floating (rasping) the sharp points off cheek teeth is one of the most common tasks a veterinarian performs.

these teeth is to crop grass when grazing.

In the back of the mature horse's mouth are 24 grinding teeth or molars—12 on top and 12 on the bottom. Between the incisors and the grinding teeth is a space where the bit rests that is called the interdental space. Males have four canine teeth or tushes that appear in the interdental space. (Females usually do not have canine teeth.) Two wolf teeth can appear in the upper jaw of the male or female horse just in front of the molars. In other words, a male horse can have 40-42 teeth, depending on the presence of wolf teeth. A female can have 36-38 teeth, also depending on the presence of wolf teeth.

Examining the teeth can tell the experienced horseman several things. It reveals the horse's age. The teeth might show evidence of cribbing. Once in a great while, a "bishoped" horse might be seen, wherein the teeth have been drilled by a dishonest trader in an attempt to make the teeth look younger.

Dentistry is an important part of equine practice, and veterinarians who treat horses do a lot of it. We will now consider the more common dental problems that occur in horses.

Parrot Mouth: This condition is due to shortness of the lower jaw. It is also called overbite, brachygnathia, rabbit tooth, or buck tooth. The horse is born with this condition and it is often inheritable. The degree of parrot mouth varies and has been classified as quarter-, half-, three-quarter-, and full-tooth overbite. The horse with a severe overbite cannot graze properly and is a poor keeper. The worst cases have to be destroyed. Milder cases get by, but should not be kept for breeding purposes because of the inheritable factor. Many horses fail in conformation classes because of parrot mouth.

To check a horse's incisor teeth, simply spread the lips slightly and examine the bite with the jaws closed. The biting edges of the incisors should meet evenly. One point worth mentioning is that some foals have a tendency for the upper lip to protrude, giving a parrot mouth appearance. However, when the teeth are checked, they may be normal. Foals, especially of certain bloodlines, will sometimes outgrow mild cases of overbite.

Undershot Jaw (Prognathia): This condition is the opposite of parrot mouth. The lower jaw is too long, and the lower incisors protrude beyond the uppers. It is not a common fault. The outcome of this problem varies with its severity, just the same as parrot mouth.

Wolf Teeth: Some horses have a small extra tooth just in front of the first premolar called a "wolf tooth." Don't confuse it with the normal tusk that is in the interdental space. The wolf tooth interferes with the bit and is, therefore, removed. Once in a while, other extra teeth may be found anywhere in the mouth, and these, too, should be extracted.

Caps: Caps are baby teeth that remain attached to the permanent teeth as they erupt. They interfere with chewing. Usually these caps are on the molars and cannot be seen. When the veterinarian finds caps, he removes them with special instruments. But most caps fall off by themselves.

Points: The most common dental procedure that equine practitioners are called on to perform is floating (rasping) points off the cheek teeth. What causes these points? Well, we already explained how a horse's tooth continually grows. Where a tooth is not evenly met by the opposite tooth, and therefore worn down, it will grow out into a sharp point. These points are very common, especially in older horses, and interfere with chewing. They are removed by a few strokes with a dental rasp, called a "float." Proper floating requires skill and it is important not to overdo it. Excessive rasping can interfere with the grinding of the feed.

Shear Mouth: This is an exaggerated example of points as described above. The spear-like points are so severe that they must first be cut off with special instruments and then rasped smooth.

Step Mouth: Here, one or more of the cheek teeth is much longer than the others, giving a step-like appearance to the molars. A molar will grow out excessively if the opposite tooth is missing or, for any reason, it is not worn down evenly with the other teeth. The projecting teeth must be cut off. In all of these conditions caused by improper or unequal wear, the condition will recur, so that repeated treatments are necessary.

Wave Mouth: In wave mouth, the biting surface of the teeth, instead of being level, undulates to form one or more "waves." Mild cases are common and need regular floating only. Severe cases are very difficult to help.

Smooth Mouth: Very old horses can have the grinding surface of the cheek teeth worn smooth. Nothing can be done to correct such teeth. Don't confuse this type of smooth mouth with the 12-year-old horse that has lost the cups in his incisor teeth and is also said to be smooth-mouthed.

Decay: Yes, a horse's teeth can decay, and caries (cavities) are the result of decay. In horses, decay is most often associated with alveolar periostitis.

Alveolar Periostitis (infection of the tooth socket): This nearly always occurs in the cheek teeth. Undernourished and wormy young horses are prone to this disease. The teeth hurt, especially when the horse drinks cold water. If the upper teeth are involved, the infection might extend up into the sinuses, and an odorous nasal discharge will be found. The infection sometimes forms a fistula, which is a draining tract on the outside of the face. The involved teeth are painful and sometimes loose.

The only treatment is to remove the diseased teeth. As you can imagine, the extraction of such a tooth is quite an involved procedure. Often the veterinarian must cut a window in the bone overlying the root of the tooth and, with a mallet and special punch, force the tooth out of its socket. Dentistry of this type is done under anesthesia, of course.

Other less common dental problems

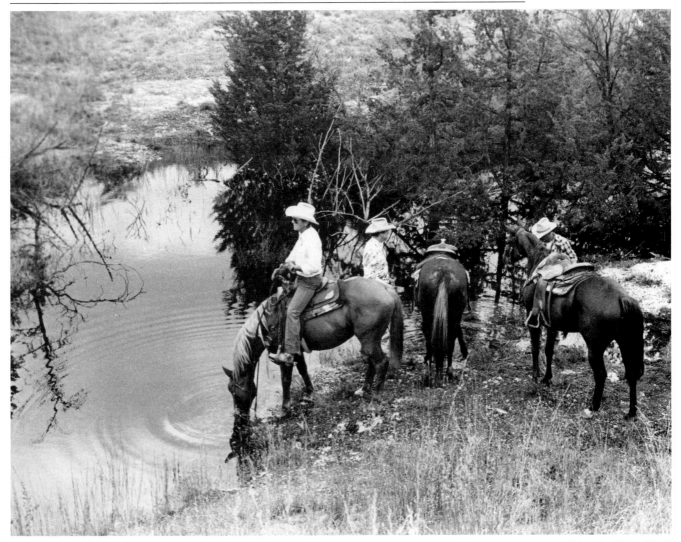

Photo by W. A. Ward

include impacted teeth, fractures of the teeth and jaw, and rare tumors and cancers of the tooth, jawbone, or gum.

The horse with dental trouble may at first show little evidence other than a loss in weight because he has trouble chewing. Later, he will cock his head, spill food from his mouth, and obviously have difficulty in eating. Every horse should have his teeth examined at least once a year. A good time to do this is when he is wormed or vaccinated.

Very old horses with worn-out mouths will die because of their faulty teeth. Sometimes they simply starve to death. In other cases the cause of death is intestinal obstruction with unchewed forage. Such horses can often be kept alive by feeding *rolled* grain and chopped hay mixed with molasses or ground pelleted hay. Frequent light feedings are best. To a human, loss of teeth is an inconvenience; to a grazing animal, it is a disaster.

Exercise

The science of horse husbandry covers many areas. These include nutrition, stabling, grooming, parasite control, vaccinations, schooling, and exercise. In most of these areas, horsemen are making great progress—keeping up with technical advances and employing new techniques. However, in the last named area, *exercise,* we seem to be weakening.

Too many horse owners are too busy doing other things to have time to exercise their horses properly. Without a good exercise program, a training schedule is incomplete. The horse that is not kept in proper condition with a good exercise schedule cannot perform his best, and is more likely to be injured.

In the wild state, on open range, or in a large pasture, the horse grazes and is almost always in motion. Moving as he grazes exercises his muscles. Actually, such a horse expends more muscular energy each day than does a show horse confined to a box stall and "exercised" for 20 minutes once a day. The free horse will also run and play, buck, roll, and otherwise maintain his muscle tone.

Since most of our pleasure horses are kept in stalls or confined to small corrals or paddocks, it is important for them to be exercised properly and sufficiently.

Exercise is beneficial in many ways. It increases the lung capacity and endurance. It strengthens the heart and blood vessels. It increases muscular strength, and preserves the elasticity of tendons and ligaments. It supples the joints. Horses are tall animals and without exercise the blood will stagnate in the lower legs. This causes the legs to "stock up," a condition known technically as edema. The well-exercised horse is less bored. He works off excess energy and is therefore much less likely to develop such vices as cribbing, weaving, or pawing.

If a horse is exercised sufficiently every day, he is less likely to develop azoturia. This is a serious and common muscle disease in show horses that are overfed, confined to a stall, and insufficiently exercised.

The horse receiving lots of daily exercise is also much less susceptible to laminitis (founder), even if he is being fed a diet high in concentrates.

Not all horses require the same *amount* or same *kind* of exercise. A pregnant mare needs plenty of exercise every day, but I do not recommend exercise for such a mare that would cause her to be excessively winded or overheated. On the other hand, a race horse needs to have his wind taxed almost daily for him to achieve optimum pulmonary efficiency.

The type of work done by a horse often determines the kind of exercise he needs. Some horses require great strength in their hindquarters for their particular use. Several examples include stock horses, cutting horses, rope horses, hunters, and jumpers. Hill climbing (if you live in a hilly area) is an excellent way to develop the muscles of the hindquarters in such horses.

In other events, such as trail and pleasure, power in the hindquarters is not essential. Thus we see that the type of exercise and its intensity is variable.

After many years of hearing me preach against starting horses too young and pushing them too hard, some of my clients decided to not ride until their horses reached the third year. Instead, they longed them one to two hours a day. Know what happened? These colts got just as sore and lame as the ones that were ridden prematurely.

Longeing should always be regarded as a method of schooling, not as a method of exercise. That means that five to fifteen minutes a day is enough. On a longe line a horse can be taught all kinds of things, including collection. Many trainers teach a horse nearly all the basics in the longeing ring. That's fine.

Why not use longeing as a form of exercise? Because at a trot or faster gait, it puts a lot of stress on the legs. At any speed faster than a walk, a horse must lean inward to maintain his balance in a relatively small circle. Meanwhile, his feet are hitting level ground. Think what that does to the joints. His foot is level, and his legs slant inward. Try running around in a small circle, flat-footed, yourself. Feel the stress in your ankle? Now, if the ring sloped inward toward the center, like a motorcycle track or an indoor human track, then perhaps longeing could be safely used for long periods of exercise.

How can you safely exercise a horse too young to ride? In large pastures, young horses tend to keep themselves exercised adequately, but we don't all have large pastures, and the demands of the show ring are such that harder muscling is needed, and that means forced exercise. If you can't ride the young horse and you can't longe him, how can you exercise him without damaging his legs? We can't all afford an equine swimming pool.

Well, you can pony a young horse. Ride an older horse and pony (lead) the youngster alongside. Go for a ride out in the country this way, or around the neighborhood. Ponying outside also has other advantages. With the older horse as his "security blanket," the young horse learns to cross water, scramble up and down dirt banks, and to pick his way through brush and down timber. He also gets used to barking dogs and kids on motorbikes. All of this will pay off later when you begin riding him outside.

Another alternative to longeing is the treadmill. Several are commercially available. Yes, they are expensive, but it's expensive to ruin the legs of a good horse, too.

The treadmill, causing the horse to labor up an inclined plane, stresses the horse's heart, lungs, and muscles, but at a walk, on a resilient surface, and in a straight line. It is much less likely to break down a colt than endless longeing or driving or riding in a small circle. A daily workout on a treadmill is like growing up in a hillside pasture for a young horse.

If you have a hillside pasture you can encourage horses of any age to walk up and down the hills endlessly by putting half the feed at the top of the hill, and half at the bottom; or their feed at the top and their water at the bottom, or vice versa.

Regardless of the exercise method, all of them, including the treadmill and ponying, can be overdone. Young horses whose legs have not matured and hardened cannot stand the same amount of hard work as a mature horse without risk of bone or joint damage. Always try to analyze what nature intended, and then use common sense in management procedures. Remember that prolonged slow exercise, like walking, is less damaging than sudden severe exercise, like speed, sharp turns, or sudden starts and stops.

The automatic hot walker is a safe, although boring method of exercising a horse, if it's used at a walk, for a long-enough period of time, on a resilient ground surface, and in both directions.

Can exercise harm a horse? I don't think so, providing the horse is a good physical specimen, is in good condition for the type of exercise he is receiving, and the exercise is not excessive. I once asked the owner of an outstanding endurance horse how he trained him (a mature Arabian stallion) so he could complete a 100-mile ride in such remarkably good condition. He told me that he rode the horse an average of 35 miles daily.

Of course, this was an exceptional horse; but in general, any *sound* horse can tolerate many miles of daily riding (walk, trot, and lope) on good, smooth resilient ground with no trouble. In fact,

he will benefit by such a program.

Note that I did not advocate sprinting, galloping on hard ground, or a lot of jumping, roping, cutting, etc. These strenuous activities can cause injuries due to concussion or strain. Let me use an analogy. A football player is not likely to injure himself in a program of cycling, jogging, calisthenics, and weight lifting. But in the game, where the player is subjected to high-speed turns, violent contact, and severe falls, injuries are common. So it is with horses.

Please note that I also said exercise could not harm "a good physical specimen." Exercise might harm a horse with faulty conformation, who is fatigued, senile, or has a disease problem.

Let me offer a tip: Keep horses in roomy corrals and keep salt at one end of each corral and water at the other. Then feed at two other locations. During the course of the day, the horses continually move from water to the feed area, then to the salt, and so on. This helps in keeping the horses legged up, especially if corrals are on a hillside.

I'll conclude with one more bit of advice. One of the most common causes of injury that I see in show horses is the policy of turning out a horse normally confined to a stall. A horse kept in a stall and fed generously is bored and bursting with energy. If he is turned loose into an arena or corral, he will usually race around, buck, and kick violently, especially if he has a lot of "hot blood." Because his body is cold, he will often injure himself.

No human athlete will enter a race or other event without first warming up to limber the muscles and joints and stimulate circulation. An equine athlete requires the same consideration. So don't turn a cold horse loose to run. Warm him up first by leading, longeing, or otherwise limbering him up. Also be particularly careful about turning out a stall-confined horse when the ground is slippery or wet.

Feeding

For many years, I have said that the practice of feeding excessive quantities of grain to young, growing horses caused bone disease. Horse owners, in

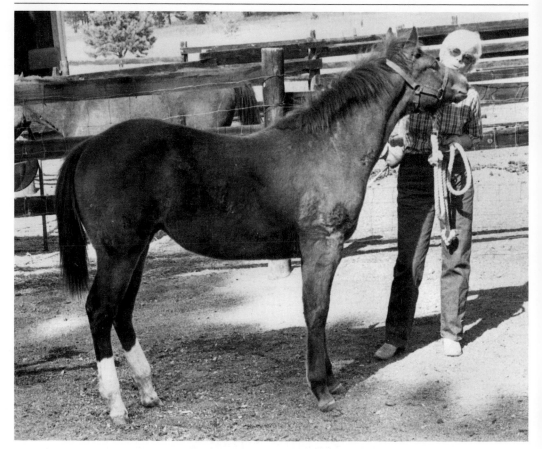

Too much grain causes contracted tendons in young horses, as seen in the cocked ankle here.

their desire to achieve maximum growth as rapidly as possible, feed foals too well, striving for success in the show ring, the sales ring, and at the racetrack.

Epiphysitis, OCD (osteochondritis dissicans), and contracted tendons have become all too common in weanlings and yearlings. Some cases are so severe that the foals have to be destroyed. Others survive, but with permanently damaged joints, abnormally straight pasterns, and a predisposition to degenerative joint disease before middle age.

In recent years, several published articles have alerted breeders to the dangers of excessive feeding. Some have taken heed, and, in my practice at least, we are finally seeing a drop in the epidemic of metabolic bone disease caused by overfeeding. For years we have cautioned breeders not to exceed one-half pound of grain per hundred pounds of body weight daily. Yet, some sources of information, including some university publications, still recommend feeding twice that amount of grain, and some even advocate free-choice grain to weanlings.

The mechanism of how excessive

grain actually damages growing bone has been described in a scientific paper, "A Dietary Etiology for Osteochondrotic Cartilage," by two scientists from the University of Maryland, Doctors T.H. Belling and M.G. Glade. I knew Dr. Belling when I was a student in veterinary school at Colorado State University. He was a horseman even back then, and we once worked a roundup together on the Wyoming border.

The Maryland paper describes an experiment in which weanling foals were deliberately fed excessive diets. At intervals, biopsy specimens were taken from the cartilage growth plates in their legs. The specimens were analyzed and studied. The results showed that feeding weanlings diets rich in grain, energy, and protein triggered changes in the chemical composition of the skeleton.

In the scientists' own words, "The findings of this study support the hypothesis that the ingestion of grain-rich meals by weanling horses is related to subsequent osteochondrotic changes in the biochemical composition of both articular and growth plate cartilages. The relative speed with which these changes occurred (appearing within three months) further emphasizes the sensitivity of growing equine cartilage to dietary influences, including excesses."

In plain English, too much grain damages bone growth, something that I have been preaching for over 20 years.

This paper, published in the *Journal of Equine Veterinary Science* (Volume 6, Number 3, 1986), along with other recent studies, will do a lot to discourage excessive grain feeding and will contribute to a better understanding of equine nutritional needs.

Here again are my recommendations for feeding weanlings and yearlings:

THE WEANLING

Foals may be weaned at any age and raised to healthy maturity, but it's best to wait until they are at least four months old. All weanlings need roughage, plus a milk supplement if under six months of age. In addition, feed one-half pound of grain per 100 pounds of body weight daily, divided into two feedings. In other words, a 400-pound weanling would get one pound of grain twice daily. The grain can be a commercial mix, or you can use rolled oats or barley. The feeding instructions on some sacks of grain advise feeding more grain than I do, but to do so increases the probability of the foal developing epiphysitis and other bone damage, and contracted tendons.

A vitamin-mineral supplement is okay, but only use one product, and follow the instructions on the label. Regional deficiencies in some geographic areas may make mineral supplementation important.

Copper and zinc are believed to play a role in developmental bone disease, so use a supplement that includes these and other trace minerals in proper proportions.

Weanlings may even be conditioned to show at halter on such a diet. A balanced pelleted hay ration, free of grain, may be fed free choice along with the above grain rations and some milk supplement. If hay pellets are fed, no hay is necessary. I like to raise halter foals on free-choice pellets and no hay. It makes a smaller belly and you can get the foal fat without having to feed excessive grain.

THE YEARLING

The yearling needs ample roughage, plus one-half pound of concentrate (grain) per 100 pounds of body weight daily. As they mature, some yearlings will require a little more concentrate. Others will require less. But again, use caution because too much grain can also cause epiphysitis and contracted tendons in yearlings. A milk supplement will help ensure adequate protein and mineral levels.

Pellets

Pelleted livestock rations have been in widespread use for a long time. Pelleted feeds for horses are more recent, and at first, many horse owners were negative toward feeding pellets. They felt that the pellet was "unnatural" and that horses required bulky rations. Time and experience have shown that horses do very well on pelleted feeds, and their use is now very widespread, with many horses subsisting entirely on such rations.

After more than 20 years of experience, it may be a good idea to review the pros and cons of feeding pelleted feeds, especially since the trend seems to be in that direction and since it is highly probable that in another 20 years, a majority of the horses in the United States will be on that kind of feed.

Pelleted feeds are simply ordinary horse feeds that are processed in feed mills and compressed into small "bite-size" pellets and sold either in bulk, or put up in sacks for ease of handling.

Many feed companies now produce pelleted horse feeds. Some of these pellets contain only hay. Others contain hay plus concentrates, and many have added minerals and vitamins and various conditioners. So some pellets are simply small "bales" of hay and are often called "hay replacer" pellets. Others are a complete balanced ration for the horse, needing no other feeds or supplements to complement them, and some companies vary the formula so the pellets can be fed to idle horses, or horses requiring extra nutrition under the demands of hard work, growth, pregnancy, or lactation.

Assuming that the pellets are being produced by a reliable firm that utilizes good quality basic feeds, and understands equine nutrition, there are many advantages to feeding pellets. Please understand that I am discussing a *complete* pellet—one containing roughage (hay), concentrates (grain, etc.), and

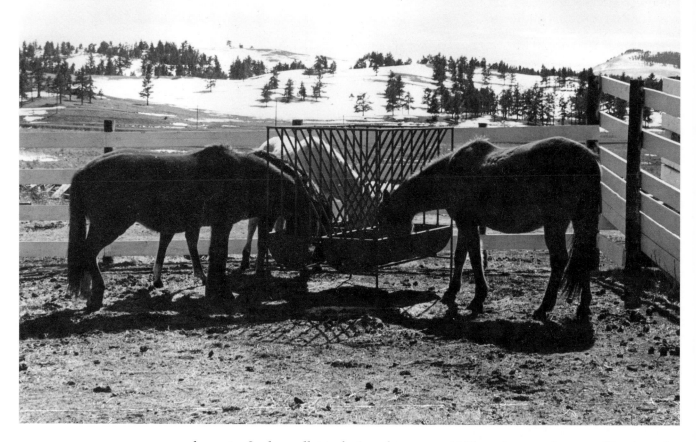

supplements. Such a pellet is designed to be the *sole* source of food for the horse. No other feed of any kind is to be offered. The horse subsists on the pelleted ration and water, with salt offered free choice on the side.

Advantages are:

1/ The ration can be accurately measured, and the contents are consistent and uniform. This virtually eliminates problems and diseases such as colic, founder, and azoturia due to feeding errors. Naturally, the pellets must be fed according to the manufacturer's directions.

2/ Pellets are convenient. They are simple to transport and to store. They take up very little room in the barn. For horses going to shows or rodeos, all you have to do is stick a sack of pellets in your trailer or truck. Your horse doesn't have to experience a feed change.

3/ There is no waste. Pellets fed in a good, tight manger or in a feed bucket are all consumed. By contrast, a noticeable percentage of hay is usually scattered and trampled.

4/ There is a maximum utilization of the ingredients in a pellet. It is nearly all digested and the horse passes very small quantities of manure. On an ordinary diet, a great deal of hay and grain passes through a horse undigested. Pelleting also tends to destroy weed seeds and mold spores due to heat generated during compression.

5/ The horse keeps a trim belly. Even when he is fed heavily enough to be fat, his bottom line is level. You see no hay bellies on pellet-fed horses. Older broodmares recover their shapes. Young horses can be put into show shape without excessive graining.

6/ There is no dust. Coughing is eliminated, and horses with heaves are benefited. Pellets don't mold unless they get wet. People with allergies will enjoy handling pelleted feeds.

7/ Horses feel great when fed a good pellet ration properly. Many large farms are now feeding pelleted feeds to all their horses. There is no hay on any of these places.

8/ Pellets are safer to feed than baled

hay and grain. The horse that gets into the feed room is unlikely to founder by overeating. You can say good-by to hay bales full of weeds, mold, bits of wire, rocks, dead rabbits, and old rubber inner tubes. The fire hazard is eliminated.

9/ Old horses, and horses with bad teeth, thrive on pellets. This type of feed can mean years of additional life to many fine old horses that can no longer subsist on ordinary feed. For horses with really bad teeth, the pellets can be soaked or ground before they are fed to make them much easier to chew and digest.

Disadvantages are:

1/ The major disadvantage to pellet feeding is the tendency of horses to chew wood. As an Arizona feedman put it, "Into each life, some rain must fall." In other words, wood chewing seems to be the price one must pay for the many advantages of pellet feeding. Several theories have been advanced as to why horses on pelleted feeds chew wood. Some say the horse craves roughage. But pellets are *made* of roughage. Moreover, it was reported that in a midwestern feeding experiment, horses were maintained in perfect physical condition for two years on a concentrated balanced ration completely lacking in roughage. Apparently horses do *not* need roughage; they need nutrients.

In the experiment mentioned, horses thrived on a few handfuls of powdered nutrients daily. However, the stalls had to be constructed of stainless steel to keep the horses from eating them.

Other people feel that the horse needs to chew abrasive feed to keep his teeth worn down. One company uses cracked corn as its major concentrate to meet this end. Some feed companies have even tried adding wood chips to their pellets, thinking that some vital ingredient was lacking, and craved by the horse.

Most of these efforts have failed to solve the wood chewing problem because horses on pellets chew wood for the same reason that any horse chews wood . . . he hasn't got anything else to do. The wood-chewing vice is the result of boredom, and since pellets are consumed much more quickly than ordinary feed, the horse has more time on his hands and consequently chews more wood.

The only present answer to the problem is to construct fences, barns, and stalls of chew-proof material. One rancher, feeding pellets to his horses, cuts limbs and throws them into this corrals to minimize damage to his fences. The horses chew the limbs instead of the fences. Several people have used smooth stones in the mangers to slow down the horses' eating and keep them occupied. A Quarter Horse enthusiast in California keeps a mineral block in her corrals. It tastes better than her wooden plank fences, and her horses spend some of their idle hours working on the block.

I have noted that many horses chew wood badly when first put on pellets, and then drop the habit when they get adjusted to the new ration. In time, most horses get to like their pellets so well that they'll prefer them to standard feeds.

2/ Another possible disadvantage to pellets is that, if a horse accidentally gains access to pasture or ordinary hay, he may be in greater danger of colic. Of course, any sudden change of feed is dangerous, but this danger may be increased in horses that have been on pelleted rations, and whose stomachs and intestines have shrunk in size.

3/ There has been some talk of the danger of choking in feeding horses pelleted feeds. I have noted that there *is* a slightly greater tendency for horses to choke on pellets than on regular feeds. However, this is not a significant problem. I have been feeding pellets either entirely or as a significant portion of my horses' rations for 25 years at this writing, and have never had one of them choke. I feed my weanling foals only pellets and concentrates, and I also feed very old horses exclusively on pellets. Otherwise, I feed a mixture of pellets and hay, mainly so that my stock won't chew the fences and the barn down.

There is evidence that most horses that have choked on pellets have been deprived of water, or have been dehydrated. Fortunately, a choke on pellets is easier for the veterinarian to relieve than a choke on coarse hay, or on a carrot or apple.

4/ Pellet feeding is expensive—if you have access to home-grown hay or pasture.

However, if you are buying hay and

grain, plus supplements, you will find pellet feeding entirely practical. Pellets cost more than hay, but you must remember the lack of waste, the small amount fed, and the good results you can expect.

5/ Another disadvantage of feeding pellets is that you cannot see what goes into them. Most horse owners know good hay when they see it, but they are at the mercy of the feed company when it comes to the ingredients of a pelleted ration. That's why it is so important to buy pellets from a reputable company. Not only must we trust the integrity of the dealer, but we must also have confidence in his technical ability to properly balance the product nutritionally. For example, some years back, a midwestern company formulated a pellet, rich in concentrates, that caused a disastrous number of gas colics, many of them fatal.

Many horsemen are going to balk at pellet feeding because "it just ain't natural." Well, I'll bet that the first horseman who ever looked at a bale of hay said the same thing. We still have a lot to learn about feeding horses, but pelleted feeds are here to stay.

Fencing

Among the most frequent injuries of horses presented to the veterinarian are those caused by fences. I would like to pass on my experience along these lines and offer my opinion as to the best types of fencing material for horse corrals and pastures.

First, however, there are some general rules that should be mentioned.

1/ The larger the area in which the horse is confined, the less likely he will be to injure himself. A 100-acre pasture is safer for a horse than a 5-acre pasture, and a roomy corral is safer than a cramped corral. This rule is modified, of course, by the fencing material used. The rule applies when any given fence is considered.

2/ Well-fed horses are less prone to fence injuries. Reaching over, through, and pawing at fences to reach a bit of grass on the other side leads to many of these injuries.

3/ Any fence is less dangerous if there are no horses on the other side. Fighting,

playing, or trying to join horses across the fence leads to many injuries.

4/ Regardless of the fencing material used, the fence is safer if it is high. Low fences encourage horses to lean over and weaken or break the fence.

Now let's consider the pros and cons of some of the popular fencing materials.

1/ *Wood.* Wooden fences are popular, attractive, and in some areas relatively inexpensive. Unfortunately, we see many serious injuries from board fences. I do not like lightweight board fences because they break too easily. If boards are used, they should be two inches thick, and the posts should be massive. Such a fence is not likely to break and impale a horse if he hits it, as will a fence made of one-inch boards. Any board fence is likely to have splinters and slivers that may puncture the horse.

Unfortunately, horses will often chew wooden fences. Painting them with various solutions will minimize wood chewing, but they are not infallible, and there is some danger from them if the horse chews anyway.

Pole fences are excellent if properly constructed, but poles are prohibitively expensive in some parts of the country. Where available at low cost, they make a fine fencing material.

2/ *Electric.* Electrified smooth-wire fence is basically a good horse fence. Injuries are not common, but escapes are. Some horses will jump through the fence instead of away from it on first contact. Tall weeds can short-circuit the fence. Horses can cleverly learn to escape when the current is off. And I have heard of horses being electrocuted when exposed to a combination of too high a voltage and wet ground.

In my opinion, electric fencing is most suitable for horses when combined with some other type. For example, a wire mesh fence may be topped with a strand of electric wire.

3/ *Mesh, woven wire, and chain-link.* These fences, if properly constructed and under the right conditions, can be satisfactory. Proper construction means no less than five feet high, and stretched on posts stout enough to stand up when a horse rubs along the fence. A big horse scratching his tail or rubbing his sides along the fence after he has been unsaddled, or when he is shedding, might bend the pipe posts used to support chain link fencing—unless these posts are 3 inches in diameter or more.

In small corrals, pawing at these fences will result in torn lower wires that get caught in the shoe and pull it off. Smooth wire can cut a pastern badly. The bottom of a chain link fence will unravel when pawed, leaving sharp ends that often puncture the sole of the foot. This is most likely to happen if the fence goes down to ground level. When horses lean against mesh or link fences, the fence bulges out and cannot be restored to its original shape.

If the top of a chain link fence is left with exposed wire ends sticking up, they very frequently rip open the lower eyelids of the horse. It is better to finish the top with a pipe rail. Here again, heavy pipe must be used or it will bend under the pressure and eventually spring loose. This pipe rail should be inserted through "eye" tops on each post. No other method will hold it securely, other than welding.

In my experience, mesh and link fences are *not* satisfactory for small corrals for the reasons cited. Of course, some horses are less destructive than others, and for such horses, the fencing requirements are simpler.

4/ *Pipe fencing.* In my opinion, pipe that is welded or bolted together is one of the best horse fencing materials available. Sections of pipe fence, already assembled and ready for installation, are commercially available in many parts of the country. Three-inch pipe welded into a three-rail fence, can be painted and looks very attractive.

In general, I prefer the heavier pipe to that of smaller diameter, and I like to see the lowest rail at least two feet above the ground. Horses often get a leg caught when lying down close to a fence if the bottom rail is too low.

The main objection to a heavy pipe fence is that when a horse kicks it, such as when fighting with another horse across the fence, painful bruises to the foot, ankle, and cannon bones can often be caused. More resilient materials, including wood, are less bruising.

5/ *Barbed wire.* In the western United States, at least, more horses are still confined by barbed wire than any other kind of fencing material. It is cheap, simple, and effective for fencing in cattle. But I think that barbed wire has disfigured, crippled, and killed more good horses than all other fencing materials combined. As a veterinarian, I have seen too many ghastly wire cuts to even consider barbed wire to fence in a valued horse.

Stables

Stables are intended to shelter and protect horses. Due to inexperience of builders and many horse owners, stables are constructed with potentially dangerous features that cause injuries to horses. Wise stable construction can reduce the frequency of injuries, but horses being what they are, no stable is totally injury-proof, just as no fence is totally injury-proof.

Stable fires are rare, but when one occurs, it is a nightmare. Consideration should be given to constructing with fire-retardant materials. If the barn has a center aisle, ideally there should be a rear exit to every stall to get horses out in case of fire. Wiring should be installed by an expert, and located so horses cannot chew it. Since mice and rats might also chew wiring, possibly causing a fire, it's safest to put wiring in conduit.

Ideally, hay and straw should not be stored in the stable. If a blaze erupts, they add fuel to the fire. Also, hay that is damp when baled can burst into flames days later from spontaneous combustion. And this has happened. So if at all possible, store hay and straw elsewhere, and keep just a few bales at a time in the stable. Many people simply stack hay and straw outside on a platform and cover it with a tarpaulin.

Of course, smoking should never be allowed near hay or bedding.

Stable alleyway floors must be made of a non-slippery material. Smooth-finished concrete or blacktop is dangerous. Rough-finished floors are available. Some horse owners simply use the natural dirt floor, sprinkling it occasionally to control any dust. A finished floor is easier to keep clean, however.

Stall doorsills should be buried below ground level, or at least constructed with rounded contours. A horse crossing a sharp, square-cornered sill can strike the point of the fetlock and fracture the sesamoid bone. Or, a blow to the coronet can cause a painful injury that sometimes leads to permanent complications.

Be sure that ceilings, the tops of doorways, and rafters are high enough that a rearing horse cannot strike the top of his head. Many horses have been "scalped" when going through low doorways. A tall horse can easily rear and hit his head against a rafter eight or nine feet high. Similarly, beware of low eaves on the outside of the barn. A horse tied outside the barn may be frightened and pull back or rear up and strike low eaves or a roof beam. Such protruding hazards can injure a careless rider, too.

Doorways and gates should always be as wide as is practical. This lessens the danger of a horse charging through a narrow doorway and hitting a shoulder or a hip against the doorpost or gatepost. This type of injury is the most common cause of "sweenied" shoulders and "knocked-down" hips in horses.

Stalls should be as large as possible to minimize the chances of a horse casting himself. The traditional 10x10 stall is simply too small for many of our larger horses, and consideration should be given to making stalls 12x12 or even larger.

(A "cast" horse is one who is lying down in such a position that he cannot get up, or one who has rolled and become stuck while on his back. The latter position is very dangerous as horses cannot lie on their backs very long without suffering internal complications that can result in death.)

Stalls should be constructed of materials that are safe, durable, and that will require the least maintenance. Wood has always been popular, but remember that many horses will chew wood. If wood is used it should be heavy enough to withstand kicking and smooth enough to prevent splinters from penetrating the horse.

The inside of a stall can be lined with ¾-inch plywood kick boards. Horses are especially fond of chewing California redwood, so although it is beautiful and durable, it is not recommended for stable construction. Wood may be lined with malleable sheet metal. In fact, some of the prefabricated portable stalls now being sold are constructed of sheet metal over wood and I think they are excellent.

Masonry barns are good in many ways, but they can cause severe abrasions if a horse is cast in a masonry stall, and horses can kick a hole in some kinds of masonry, such as concrete block.

All-metal barns work well, if adequately lined and insulated, and if the construction is sturdy enough.

The choice of materials for stall floors varies widely, and is quite controversial. I have seen almost everything used: wood, plastic, concrete, asphalt, rubber matting, and various types of soil. In my part of the country (southern California), we like a compacted floor of decomposed granite. If concrete is used, it should have a drain, and should have an extremely deep layer of bedding on top of it to minimize chances of the horse slipping and falling. And it should be a rough-finished concrete.

Clay is a popular material for stall floors, but clay and other types of soil require periodic refilling where horses dig holes in it. Regardless of the material used for stall floors, it should provide good drainage and sanitation. Straw or shavings should be used for bedding, but beware of using moldy straw; if a horse eats it, he might get sick. *Never* bed a stall with sand. Too many horses get sand colic this way.

Stall walls should be solid at least halfway up. When a partial partition (such as pipe or spaced boards) is used, a horse can stick a leg through and get it hung up. For the upper half of the stall walls, you can either continue with a solid partition or use something like chain-link fencing, wire mesh, metal bars, etc. Total separation (via a solid partition) minimizes fighting and exposure to respiratory diseases; but horses are usually happier if they can see their neighbors and look out into the alleyway or outdoors, instead of being kept in "solitary confinement." Using something like chain link, etc., also increases air circulation, which keeps stalls cooler in hot weather.

When possible, it is convenient for each stall to have an electric light, but it should be high enough so a horse can't reach it, and protected by some type of metal guard. Horses have been known to munch on light bulbs.

Some horse owners use heat lamps in the winter to help keep summer coats on their horses, or to take the chill out of foaling or "sick-room" stalls. If heat lamps are used, make sure the stable wiring is adequate to carry this increased electrical load. Also place heat lamps out of reach of the horse.

Some heat lamps are adjustable, and in one case a horse "adjusted" his heat lamp so it was pointing straight up to the hayloft floor . . . just inches away. Because the heat from the lamp was so intense, the wood in the floor was actually smoldering when discovered. In another case, a heat lamp set a horse's blanket on fire. And a heat lamp can set bedding on fire. So be very careful when using these lamps.

The inside of the stalls should be clean, smooth, and free of all dangerous protrusions such as nails, bolts, latches. If a stall has an automatic waterer, it should either be recessed or guarded with a smooth pipe rail to prevent damage to both waterer and horse. If buckets or tubs are used for feed and water, they should be fastened to the wall, so the horse can't get his feet tangled in them, and they should be free of sharp, jagged edges. Help keep the water supply clean by placing it as far as possible from where you feed the hay and grain.

Regarding mangers, I prefer them to be wide (24 to 30 inches), long (full width of the stall), and deep (chest high to the horse). Slope the side facing the horse down to a foot-wide, poured concrete floor. The slope prevents the horse from bumping his knees. If you use a wood floor for the manger, inspect it frequently for splinters. Such a manger prevents hay from being scattered all over the stall, and is easy to clean. It's even easier to clean if you leave about an inch of space between the manger floor and one side; then you can sweep out chaff, etc.

The manger can be divided into compartments for salt, grain, and hay.

To save time when feeding, build the manger so hay and grain can be put in without opening the stall door. If you feed from the alleyway, put a little trap door in the wall partition above the manger; or if you feed from the hayloft, put a trap door above the manger in the hayloft floor.

Also build the manger so it has no sharp edges. If it is constructed of wood,

the edges can be covered with sheet metal to prevent wood chewing.

Don't forget to include a good-size feed room and tack room in your stable. Novices often forget these when drawing their plans. How big the feed room should be depends on whether you will keep hay in it, and how much. If you just keep grain in it and a few miscellaneous tools, a small one will be fine. You will not be happy if you keep tack and feed in the same room, because your equipment will always be covered with dust.

Since tack thefts are a big problem, it's safest not to have a window in the tack room, and the door should be sturdy and built so it can be securely locked.

Ideally, each stall should open into a separate paddock or corral. This allows horses a little bit of exercise; and if horses are separated, it is easier to control their diets, and will minimize their fighting, which often results in serious injuries.

Something else to keep in mind: If two horses share the same stall and corral, and if both try to go in or out of the stall door at the same time, this can result in a knocked-down hip or sweenied shoulder. For this reason, when two or more horses share the same stall, the doorway should be extra-wide, or the stalls should simply be open on one side, with no doorway at all.

Stall doors should open away from the horses so they are less likely to get caught in a partially opened door. This causes *many* serious injuries. If you build Dutch doors, the bottom door should be high enough (at least four feet) to discourage a horse from thinking about jumping over it. If Dutch doors are left open so a horse can go in and out at will, secure both doors so they stay open. A horse can be injured when the top door blows shut and he tries to go under it; or if the bottom door is partially open, and he tries to go in or out of the stall.

The stall door latches should not have any protruding bolts or sharp handles. Beware of welded horseshoe latches; I know of many horses that caught their lower jaws inside a horseshoe and fractured their jaws severely. If you want to use horseshoe latches, use small pony shoes, or weld a bar across the shoe to

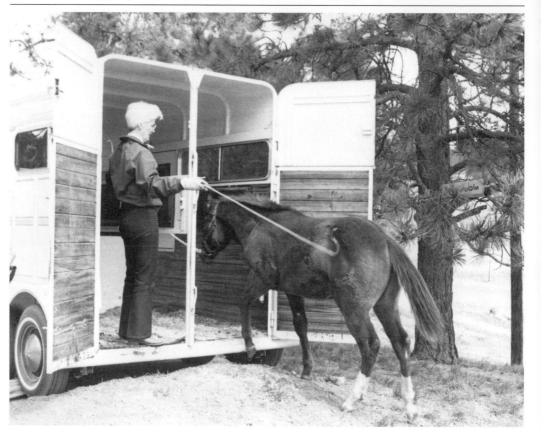

The time to train for trailer loading is when you are not in a hurry. Another cardinal rule is that you can't control the horse if you can't control your own temper.

prevent a horse from sticking his lower jaw through it.

Building a stable properly takes experience and ingenuity. Before you build, show your plans to your veterinarian. He has seen hundreds of barn-caused injuries, and he might be able to offer some suggestions to make yours a safer stable.

Trailering

In more than 30 years of horse practice, I have seen countless victims of trailer accidents. Most of the accidents could have been prevented.

There were the gruesome results of a horse's foot going through the floorboards, and being ground off on the highway. Obviously, sound floorboards could have prevented such disaster.

Then there are the trailers that break loose from the towing vehicle, a tragedy preventable with a good, secure hitch. I remember the time I personally drove off with my hitch unlatched. Fortunately, the trailer detached at low speed before I hit the highway, with no harm done except damage to my trailer tongue. That mishap could have been prevented by inspecting the hitch, a procedure that

should be done every time you move the trailer.

I thought about the colts and a few grown horses that have climbed up into the trailer manger. I had a weanling mule foal, in fact, who managed to get all four feet into the manger and his head out the front window. Of course, being a mule, he didn't injure himself, but this kind of accident is preventable by putting a bale in the manger.

I recall the Arabian stallion that cast himself upside down in a trailer. He was tied in with a chain and the frantic owners could not release him. Fortunately, we were able to cut his nylon halter with a sharp knife, and he escaped without injury. Prevention? Slip knots, accessible from outside the trailer compartment, plus safety snaps, such as the panic snaps.

I have seen hundreds of coronet wounds and leg injuries in trailered horses. Protective bandages and boots would have prevented most of them.

Of course, I remember the many accidents I have been called to. Most of these could have been avoided by sensible driving. Whether or not a trailer is behind the car, excessive speed causes most accidents. People drive too fast, turn too abruptly, stop or accelerate too suddenly, and change lanes too sharply. Interestingly, I noticed that when the 55 mph speed limit was introduced, I saw fewer trailer wrecks.

A lot of injuries are due to faulty equipment. Hind legs get over butt ropes or bars placed too low; unpadded butt chains abrade hind ends and tail heads; loose dividers, tail gates, and sidewalls entrap feet. Good maintenance and common sense can prevent most injuries.

Many accidents occur when the trailer is not in motion. People tie horses to trailers that aren't attached to a vehicle. The horse pulls back and the trailer starts to chase the horse. *Big trouble!* Or, the horse is tied too long to the trailer, and gets a foot over the tie rope. Or, the horse is tied to a part of the trailer where a sharp-edged license plate, or projection of some sort, lacerates the horse.

Yes, I can remember many, many trailer-related injuries, most of them preventable if common sense, caution, and good management procedures had been used. But, all of the accidents I have mentioned, added together, plus all of those I have forgotten, are insignificant in numbers if compared with one type of trailer-related injury: *the loading accident.*

Yes, by far the most common cause of injury to horses, and often to the people involved, greatly outnumbering all other causes, is the act of loading a horse into a trailer.

Horses, while being loaded, fly back and bash their heads on the tops of the trailers. If they are tied or snubbed, halters or ropes may break, causing the horse to fall over backwards. Skulls or necks may fracture. Many horses are ruined or killed this way. Flying back out of a trailer, or backing away from the ramp, whirling away, or turning in the trailer in an attempt to escape causes many mutilating injuries to horses. Rearing up while resisting loading has caused more head and face lacerations than I can possibly remember.

An inept attempt to load a horse into a trailer causes not only physical injury to the horse, but psychological scarring as well. Many such horses are permanently terrified of trailers.

How do you prevent such injuries? *Train the horse to load and to haul properly.* Easily said, but rarely done. So, I think the most useful contribution I can make to this issue is to pass on the best loading techniques I have observed in a lifetime of working with horses. There are two of them. No claims for originality are made, but these are the best methods I know to teach a horse to load into a trailer happily.

METHOD ONE: Start the day the horse is foaled. Load mare and foal into a trailer. Pet the foal. Unload them. Repeat this a couple of times. Do it daily until the foal looks forward to the procedure. It is easy at this age. As soon as the foal is nibbling grain, reward the loading with a little sweet feed. After a while, start to drive around *slowly.* Teach the foal that trailering is a part of life.

METHOD TWO: For those who waited too long to use Method One, position the trailer in a pasture or corral so that it cannot roll, tip, or jiggle. For trailers lacking a ramp, it may help to put the wheels in a small trench to lower the height of the trailer floor. Feed the horse in the trailer and nowhere else. Start feeding on the trailer floor, and gradually move the feed towards the manger. Feed from both sides of a two-horse trailer. In a few weeks, the horse will *love* the trailer.

There are other good methods available and there are also some videotapes done by top trainers that show how you can train your horse to load quietly and safely. Most of the methods gradually build a conditioned response in the horse to move forward, on either side of the trainer, and then use that response to load the horse. They teach the horse to see the trailer as a sanctuary.

In my experience with horses that are *really* bad to load, most of the methods usually advocated won't work, and often lead to disastrous accidents. I'm referring to such methods as war bridles, snubbing the horse to the manger, using butt ropes, and attaching ropes to the front feet and advancing them one foot at a time.

To sum up, the vast majority of trailer-related accidents I have seen were caused during attempts to load the horse. Therefore, the most important single safety precaution one can take to avoid injury is to be sure that the horse is properly trained to load.

41

Spaying

Traditionally, mares, because of their breeding value, have only been spayed to correct physical or behavioral problems. For example, tumors of the ovary are not unusual in mares. Such ovaries are removed surgically. However, almost always a tumor is confined to a single ovary. Removing one ovary does not alter the mare's basic reproductive cycle, nor does it make her sterile, so such a mare is really not neutered. The same thing would be true if only one testicle were removed from the male. A stallion with one testicle is fertile and as masculine as a stallion with two testicles.

Therefore, the truly spayed mare is a mare that has had *both* ovaries surgically removed and that is nearly always done to correct behavior problems. Some mares seem to cycle constantly and are always "horsing" (in heat). They can be irritable, quarrelsome, and sometimes downright dangerous. Spaying such mares *usually* (but not always) corrects their behavior. I have known a number of fine performance mares that, once spayed, became much more docile and dependable and went on to even greater accomplishments in their athletic careers.

I have a number of questions:

Should more mares be spayed? Will spayed mares be as dependable and desirable as geldings?

I suspect that spayed mares will be every bit as good as geldings. Mares have not been neutered for centuries as stallions have, simply because it is a more complicated operation. The gonads of the stallion are in the scrotum, outside of the abdominal cavity, and are readily accessible to surgical removal. However, the ovaries of the mare are *within* the abdominal cavity, requiring a laparotomy (incision into the abdominal cavity).

One thing should be understood. When a dog or cat is spayed, a panhysterectomy is done. That is, the ovaries *and the uterus* are removed. If only the ovaries are removed, dogs and cats may develop a pyometra, which is a pus-filled uterus. In large animals, like horses and cattle, spaying may be properly performed by removing *only* the ovaries, a less drastic operative procedure.

Mares may be spayed in two ways:

1/ The vaginal approach. This operation is done with the mare standing, usually in a stocks. Local anesthesia and perhaps sedation is used. An incision is made deep in the vagina, and the ovaries are amputated, within the abdominal cavity, with a special instrument called an ecraseur.

2/ The abdominal approach. Under general anesthesia, an incision is made into the abdomen, and the ovaries are removed through this incision.

Each method has its advantages and disadvantages, and surgeons usually have preferences as to the method used.

I suspect that young fillies, at weaning age, or even much younger, could be quickly and easily spayed, and would turn out to be as reliable as performance horses as geldings are.

But I don't know this positively, because *I have never spayed a young filly.* Nobody ever asked me to in 30 years of horse practice.

I don't know of *any* veterinarian who has routinely spayed large numbers of fillies before the age of sexual maturity. If there is such a person, I would like to hear about it.

I know this: With the present supply of horses exceeding the demand, spaying fillies is an idea worth trying. It's possible that spayed fillies will develop into working horses even *better* than the traditional geldings.

Gelding

Castration is the most common equine surgical operation. In horsemen's language this operation, which consists of removing the testicles, is known as gelding, and the castrated stallion is henceforth called a gelding.

Inexperienced horsemen sometimes do not understand the reason for gelding, and there is a tendency for novices to delay gelding and keep a horse a stallion when, in fact, he should be gelded. As a result, we have a great surplus of stallions in all breeds today. Many of these inferior stallions are bred, and this practice is detrimental to the improvement of any breed.

Only the best stallions should be preserved for breeding. Any stallion that is deficient in temperament, conformation,

42

size, stamina, or performance should be culled. Breeds are improved only by breeding the best to the best.

If a stallion is unsuitable for breeding, he should be gelded for several reasons. First of all, a gelding is more tractable and easier to manage than a stallion. Oddly enough, this is the very reason many inexperienced owners do not geld their horses. They feel that there is more status to owning a stallion than owning a gelding. Many men feel that they have more *machisimo* riding or handling a stallion. They should realize that real horsemen, the top hands, prefer a gelding unless the horse has breeding potential.

The reason seasoned horsemen prefer a gelding is because, other things being equal, the gelding usually makes a using horse superior to a stallion, or even a mare.

By superior, we mean more dependable, more consistent, and more tractable. Observe that most of the records for performing horses are held by geldings. Kelso, Forego, and John Henry were great running Thoroughbred geldings. The immortal roping horse Baldy was a gelding. Nearly all the truly great jumping horses and three-day event horses are geldings. The majority of the greats in endurance riding, rodeo, and speed events are geldings. All of the old-time cow outfits used nothing but geldings, and so do modern ranches that maintain large remudas. Good geldings served the mounted police in the past, and still do. The cavalry units of the world were largely mounted on geldings.

It is probable that many of the performance records that are held by stallions would have been even more impressive if they had been geldings. But, of course, geldings have lost their value for breeding purposes.

The knowledgeable horseman does not hesitate to geld a colt. Some horses, especially of chunky or thick-set conformation, tend to get a crested neck if they are not gelded. While a massive neck is desirable in a draft horse, it is a detriment in a saddle horse. Heavy-necked horses are always heavy on the forehand, difficult to collect, and less agile than slender, graceful-necked horses.

A common misconception concerns the age at which a stallion should be gelded. Many horsemen are under the erroneous impression that a horse's testicles do not descend until he's near maturity, and that he cannot be gelded until around two years of age. A majority of American horsemen think that delaying castration will mean a larger colt, and a more muscular development. In fact, it doesn't make a bit of difference at what age a colt is gelded. In many parts of the world it is the custom to geld soon after foaling. Many of Britain's great steeplechase horses, competing in what might be the most severe athletic test in the horse world, are gelded early in life.

There are many techniques used for castrating horses. Some veterinarians do the operation with the horse standing, using a local anesthesia. But most surgeons prefer general anesthesia. A wide variety of anesthetic agents are now available for use, and some of the new short-acting anesthetics are very safe, very smooth, and free of the excitement and struggling that characterized the older anesthetic drugs. Regardless of the technique used, the object is the complete removal of *all* testicular and hormone-forming tissue.

If any hormone-forming tissue whatsoever is left behind, the horse will—although sterile—show masculine (stallion-like) behavior. Such a horse is said to be proud-cut.

A proud-cut horse is a nuisance, although in some cases he is useful for chasing and gathering wild horses, or for use as a teaser on breeding farms to detect mares in heat. Theoretically, a proud-cut horse can be operated on again, although that can actually present a very difficult surgical challenge.

Most proud-cut horses are the result of an amateur's efforts at surgery. A trained and competent veterinarian won't make this mistake because of the rather elementary anatomy involved.

Many properly castrated geldings will continue to show some degree of masculine behavior following surgery. This may include excitement and even attempts to mount a mare in heat. Such behavior does not necessarily mean that the horse is cut proud. Male hormone is secreted by other glands in the body so that even after castration, some degree of masculinity will persist. This will vary from one individual to another.

The testicle develops, before birth, within the abdomen. Later, it descends through the inguinal canal to its normal locations within the scrotum. If one testicle fails to descend, the horse is called, in medical terminology, a unilateral cryptorchid. If both testicles fail to descend, the horse is a bilateral cryptorchid.

Horsemen often call a cryptorchid horse a ridgeling, or, sometimes, an "original" horse.

If the testicle is retained within the inguinal canal, rather than in the belly proper, the term flanker or high flanker may be used.

In many horses, descent of the testicle might be delayed. A horse that is a cryptorchid at six months of age might be normal as a yearling or two-year-old. Hormone injections are often used to encourage descent of a retained testicle. Such treatment may be of value in a flanker, but is very unlikely to benefit a true abdominal cryptorchid.

Only rarely does a retained testicle descend after two years of age. Once in a while, a testicle will descend through the inguinal canal, but then, instead of progressing into the scrotum, will instead migrate out under the skin of the groin to become an ectopic testicle.

If a two-year-old horse has any of the above-mentioned forms of cryptorchidism, the following is always true.

1/ The horse should be castrated. Cryptorchidism is inheritable, and cryptorchid horses often have a bad temperament until gelded. There is also a tendency for retained testicles to develop cancer after maturity. Therefore, a mature cryptorchid must be completely gelded. If one or both testicles are retained within the belly, major abdominal surgery will be required.

2/ Testicles not within the scrotum will be sterile. The testicle cannot produce live sperm unless it is below body temperature. That is the reason the testicle is located outside the body, within the scrotum. If one testicle is cryptorchid, however, the horse can still sire foals with the normal testicle. Such horses spread this defect within their progeny.

In very rare instances, horses are born with only one testicle. Such horses, known as monorchids, can only be differentiated from unilateral cryptorchids by surgical exploration. Of course, such a defective stallion should be gelded.

In summary, colts normally have two testicles within the scrotum. If one or both glands seem to be retained, wait until the colt is two years of age before resorting to the operation (abdominal cryptorchid ectomy). Retained testicles might descend within that time.

In normal colts, decide whether the colt has potential as a breeding stallion. If the answer is no, make plans to geld him early, at least as a yearling. If the answer is maybe, delay surgery until you see how the colt turns out. If the answer is yes, then be sure you have suitable facilities for confining a stallion, and be sure you know how to handle him properly.

Horses Need Vacations

Everybody understands the need for vacations. We all need, for our mental and physical well-being, periods of rest. We require a day of rest every week to replenish our energies. Occasionally we require longer periods of rest—vacations—to recover our enthusiasm, our drive, and our strength for our everyday job.

Horses need vacations, too. Many horses are worked daily, and never have the opportunity to enjoy a vacation. I'm not thinking of the horse used for cross-country pleasure riding. This type of use does not sour a horse mentally, or deplete him physically. I'm thinking of the horse trained to do a demanding and highly specialized type of work such as reining, cutting, roping, barrel racing, or dressage. If you own a horse trained to do such work, and use him for that purpose every day, you should appreciate the value of a periodic vacation for the horse.

Sports such as those mentioned above are stressful athletic activities. They tax the horse mentally (psychologically). The horse might (and should) enjoy the activity, but these sports require concentration, and will fatigue the horse mentally, especially if overdone.

Too, these sports strain the horse physically. They stress bones, muscles, ligaments, and tendons. Inevitably, injuries occur. If the horse keeps working, healing is interfered with, and chronic

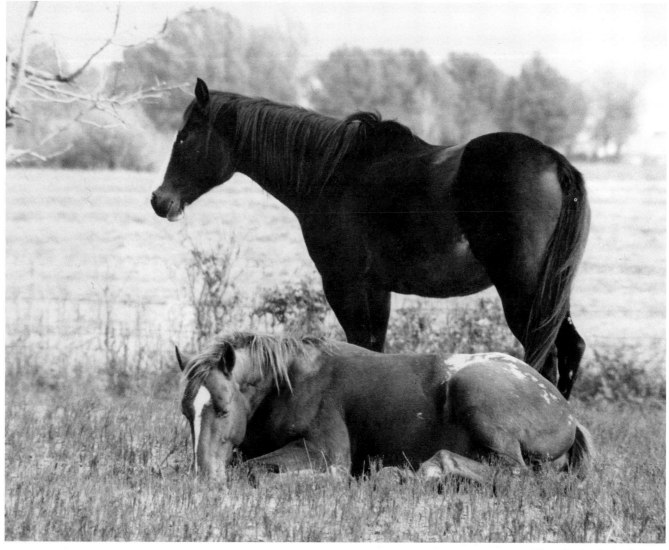

Photo by Paula Deckelman

unsoundness might eventually develop.

To help you understand the concept I am advocating, let's consider human athletes as an analogy. Does a professional ball player play every day, all year long? No. A baseball pitcher might only pitch part of a game because his arm tires, because it grows painful, or because his game is off for psychological reasons. A football player might return to the bench for the same reasons. A horse cannot tell you that he's "not with it" today, or that his back is sore, or that an old bruise is throbbing. If you're a real horseman, you'll know he's not right, and look for the cause.

Regular routines are dulling to one's sharpness. This is true of horses, as well as humans. If one is a hurdler, the training routine includes long-distance jogging, calisthenics, and sprinting, as well as actual running of the hurdles. A jumping horse should have variety in his training, too. It is damaging to ask the horse, day after day, to warm up, jump the same course in the same ring, and then cool out. The jumper, or cutting horse, or roping horse needs days of quiet riding cross-country, and periods of rest to remain alert and sharp for his event. Many riders, especially youthful riders who have lots of time and little experience, tend to overwork their horses.

A vacation of several months can be very valuable to a hard-working performance horse, especially if he is no longer young. A long lay-up refreshes his mind, and allows many minor chronic leg ailments to heal. Time is the greatest healer. A human athlete engaged in a strenuous sport will often finish the season with many injuries. He might have strained muscles, sore shins, a taped wrist, a knee in a brace, etc. Then during the off season, his injuries heal, and hopefully he's in shape for next season. If he played all year, he might soon be too unsound to perform. A horse is the same way.

It's a good idea, during such a lay-up, to pull the shoes. This gives the feet a chance to spread out and grow in a natural way for a while, uncramped by shoes. Of course, I'm assuming that the horse has normal feet that *can* be left unshod. Some horses have foot problems and require constant shoeing. Your farrier should know.

During these vacations, I'm not suggesting that your horse be confined and not allowed exercise. Not at all. If the horse is locked in a stall, or any space too small, it will not benefit him mentally or physically. A sound horse, laid up for such a vacation, should have a pasture or at least a big corral to play in. If the vacation must be in confined quarters, be sure to provide daily light exercise. The human athlete who is not in active training or competition ideally stays in shape between seasons by exercising regularly. He may run, jog, skip rope, lift weights, etc., in order to stay in shape. Similarly, a performance horse on vacation can be used for quiet trail riding interspersed with long easy canters in a ring or on good soft ground.

The Older Horse

Like people, horses in the United States are living longer than they used to, and for the same reasons: better nutrition, and better medical care.

There's no doubt in my mind that the single greatest factor contributing to the increased life span of today's horses is worm control. When I graduated from veterinary school many years ago, we had only one drug for the control of strongyles in horses, and that was phenothiazine. Not only were we limited to a single drug, but most horse owners, in fact, did not use that drug. It was best known to the breeders of race horses and those few better-informed owners who bothered to keep abreast of new developments.

Some horse owners then used chewing tobacco or garlic, in a futile attempt to worm their horses. Most people used nothing, and most horses lived out their lives perpetually parasitized. Remember that back then we only had as many horses in this country as we now have in the state of California alone. Despite that, we frequently saw horses die from vascular disease caused by bloodworm damage. Some of the horses I saw die from ruptured arterial aneurysms were only three or four years of age.

Then, as now, colic was the most common cause of death in the horse and most cases of colic then, and even now, are related directly or indirectly to bloodworm-damaged intestinal arteries.

Today, a profusion of drugs effective against bloodworms is available. More are being developed every year. Many methods of worming are available via stomach tube, oral pastes, drenches, and top dressings for feed. Most important, most horse owners today are informed.

Most horses today are companion animals, or valuable competition animals. They are valued by an interested and informed public. Horse publications disseminate a wealth of information. Horse owners are also interested in lectures, clinics, and courses. They buy books, films, and videotapes.

As a result, most horses are receiving some kind of worm control, and even if it's not optimum control, their lifetime load of bloodworms is reduced, and they suffer less blood vessel damage than did horses years ago.

Consequently, even though the horse population has increased to five times what it was when I started practice, a much lower percentage of horses are dying of parasite-caused diseases. Therefore, a higher percentage of them are living into old age to eventually die, like us, of other causes such as cancer, heart disease, and so on.

Also, since the great increase in the horse population has been in companion animals, to whom the owners become quite attached, a lot of old horses are retired nowadays, or at least semi-retired, to live out their years in peace and comfort.

Lastly, the care and management of horses has greatly improved. We see fewer barbed-wire enclosures, more stalls, and well-built paddocks. Better trailers mean fewer accidents. New vaccines prevent premature deaths from tetanus, flu, sleeping sickness, and strangles. Most horse owners understand the

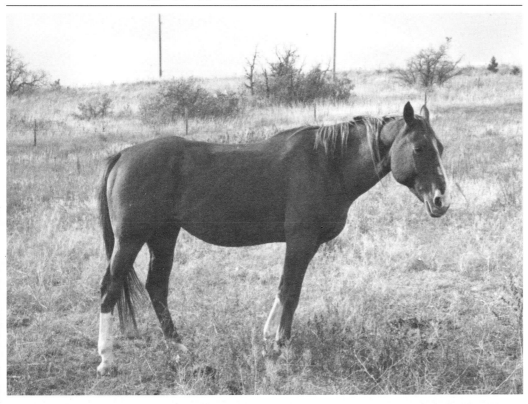

importance of dentistry, especially in the older horse. They have their horses' mouths examined, and dental problems corrected. Lots of people now request routine physical examinations for their older horses.

As a result of all of the preceding, we see a lot of old horses these days. Sound horses in their 20s, and even in their 30s, which used to be a bit unusual, are seen frequently now. There are lots of 25-year-old broodmares, nursing fine foals, and pregnant again to boot. There are lots of good working and performing horses in their late 20s and their early 30s.

Feed has made a difference, too. A lot of old horses with defective or missing teeth just couldn't make it years ago on hay or pasture. Today we have a variety of processed feeds such as chopped al-falfa, meals, and pellets, which are a boon to the old horse who can't quite chew his roughage the way he used to. Most significantly, the availability of pelleted feed has been a blessing to the equine geriatric set. Old horses thrive on pellets. Even toothless horses can gum them around until, as the pellet is moist-ened with saliva, it disintegrates. Dip a pellet in water, and see what happens to it. I recommend, for aging horses with dental insufficiencies, that a diet of pel-

lets be fed exclusively instead of hay.

An old horse can be a joy. They are usually past the foolishness and flighti-ness of youth. They are wise and de-pendable. They have learned human language, and they understand more than younger horses do. If they were not abused in their youth, they can be sound. They know their job. If they're good horses, and have been properly trained and handled, older horses are hard to beat for a wide variety of uses including pleasure riding, cow work, packing, hunting, some competitive trail riding, and many other things. There have been horses past 20 years of age that were legendary in their big league events including roping, cutting, English classes, rodeo bucking events, and so on.

Old horses, like old dogs, are the ones animal-lovers bond most closely with. We hate to lose them and so the longer we can delay that tragic point in our lives, the happier we're going to be.

So, take care of that old horse, and he should go on for many more years. Take care of his feet. Protect him from ex-tremes of weather, and from insect pests. Exercise him regularly, but don't over-work him. Spend a little time with him. Talk to him. He'll talk back.

The Last Favor

This isn't a pleasant subject and it's one seldom discussed in print. We're talking about euthanasia, usually euphemistically called "putting a horse down" or "putting him to sleep." These last two terms have been confused with anesthesia, so it's better to honestly talk about euthanasia, or simply destroying the horse.

Having to destroy a horse is a decision that, regrettably, will befall most horse owners at some point in their lives. As a veterinarian, I have had to end the lives of thousands of animals, including many hundreds of horses. After more than 30 years of practice, it is still the most difficult and most unpalatable task I am called upon to do. It is never easy, and even when I do not know the horse, it is an emotionally draining experience.

If the horse is young, I think how sad it is that it could not have had its full measure of joyful life and activity. If the horse is old, I am saddened by the thoughts of how it was once young and spirited. Often I remember the horse as a youngster, because I have seen many horses through their life cycle, from birth to death.

Veterinarians differ in their philosophies regarding the act of euthanasia, but I personally will not end the life of a horse unless I can fully justify the act because of humane reasons. When I first started practice, I did not adhere to this policy, but I have through most of my career.

For the veterinarian, the decision is not so difficult when the horse is suffering from an irreparable problem. Examples would include foals born with serious deformities, old horses suffering from terminal diseases or painful afflictions, or any horse with a hopeless disease or injury (fatal colics, certain fractures, cancer, etc.).

The decision is more difficult when the horse has a problem that is painless, or at least tolerably painful (as in a foal born blind, or a horse with advanced ringbone), but in which the problem eliminates the *use* of the horse.

Similarly, the decision is easy for some owners. If the horse cannot be used, then the *practical* thing to do is simply to painlessly end the horse's life. These people are usually objective, pragmatic persons. But for other people, ending a life, especially if it is the life of an animal to which they are attached, is a difficult and sometimes impossible decision for them to make. In such a situation, the veterinarian's sensitivity, empathy, and judgment are put to the severest test.

Nearly always, we want to do "what is best." The problem is that we vary in our perception of what is best.

I have seen hundreds of clients cling to an aging, unsound, unrideable horse because they loved it when, undeniably, the practical thing to do would have been to painlessly allow the animal to "go to sleep." I have done it myself, retiring a mare at 22 years of age, and feeding her until finally when she was 34 years of age, I did of necessity what I perhaps should have done years earlier. I have an old mule now that will probably go the same route.

Okay, I have the space for keeping an old-timer, but how about the person who has only the room or finances to keep one horse? Many times I have seen a young person who loves to ride keeping an old, unrideable horse alive and giving up their riding because they cannot make the decision to end the life of that horse.

When the necessity for euthanasia has been established, most veterinarians do it by injecting an anesthetic, rapidly and intravenously. Correctly performed, the horse is anesthetized—asleep—before he falls to the ground. However, it will take some time before death occurs. There may be some movement, and the heart may continue to beat for some time. It is important to understand, however, that the horse *is* anesthetized—unconscious—and totally unaware of what is happening.

Ranchers, usually being practical people who have witnessed the birth and death of many animals, often request that a horse be shot when it must be killed. This is, admittedly, the quickest and the most inexpensive way to end a horse's life, assuming that the bullet is properly placed in the brain.

For most owners of "pet" horses, however, the use of a gun is unaesthetic, and, especially in a suburban environment, they prefer that an anesthetic be used.

It is not pleasant to discuss how to shoot a horse, but the method is something every rider and every law enforcement officer should know and I am going to explain it here. If a horse is fatally injured in the back country, far from veterinary care, it may be necessary for the rider to destroy that animal to end its suffering, or to direct someone else how to do it. A small-caliber weapon is all that is needed. A .22-caliber handgun is adequate. Draw a line from the horse's left eye to its right ear, and from the left ear to the right eye. Where the lines intersect, on the forehead, is where the muzzle of the gun is placed. Stand back at arm's length, because, when shot, the horse will fall instantaneously, and care must be taken that the horse doesn't fall on the person holding the weapon. *But*, do not shoot from a distance. The muzzle should be right at the forehead, where the lines intersect.

Obviously, the usual precautions should be taken when handling firearms lest the tragedy of an injured horse be compounded by the accidental shooting of a human being. This is a job for a person who is familiar with the weapon being employed.

The most important thing is the accurate placement of the shot, as described. The brain of a horse, despite its large head, is only the size of a man's fist, and the bullet must enter the brain or the task will be botched.

An unpleasant subject, but, regrettably, an important one.

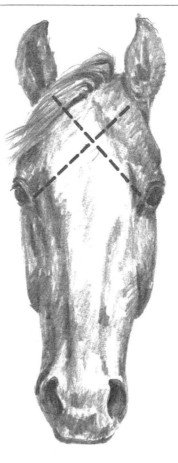

The intersection of the two lines marks the spot where you may be sure that a bullet will strike the brain.

2 ILLNESS AND INJURIES

Colic

A lot of horse owners ask, "Why do horses get colic?" They are referring, of course, to true colic, which is pain originating from the digestive tract. A horse may show colicky pain from other causes, such as a twisted uterus or kidney stones, but most colic originates from the stomach or intestines.

The horse is an incompletely evolved creature. Horses were originally small, multiple-toed swamp-dwelling animals subsisting on succulent vegetation. As his habitat dried out and converted to dry, grassy plains, the horse evolved to adapt to this new environment. He became a one-toed running animal, grazing the grass-covered prairies.

Unfortunately, the horse's digestive tract wasn't the best system for this new environment. Ruminant animals, such as cattle and sheep, that chew the cud, are far better equipped to survive on such a diet because they have a four-compartmented stomach. The grass they

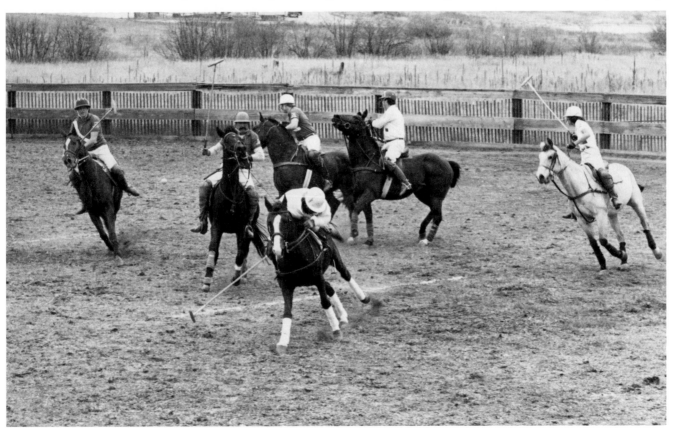

eat is regurgitated, rechewed, fermented, mixed with digestive juices, compressed, and stirred around. By the time it leaves the fourth stomach and enters the small intestine, the food is in a semi-liquid state, and easily passes through the animal.

This isn't true in horses. Horses have just one stomach, like we do. Their feed is chewed once in a semi-solid state. In fact, it comes out the other end in a similar condition; there is a lot of undigested material in horse manure. That's why birds will eat manure.

The large intestine of the horse has a very large diameter, but at certain points where it makes turns, it narrows greatly. The bulky, heavy intestinal contents in the horse contribute to obstructions and twisted intestines, and the unprocessed material easily ferments and forms gas, another cause of colic. In ruminants, most of the gas production occurs in the stomachs and is belched up. In horses, the gas is formed right in the intestine.

In addition to all this, the strongyle or bloodworm, the most common parasite of the horse, damages the intestinal arteries in its larval migrations and interferes with the blood supply to the intestines. That's why regular worming is an important part of horse management. We have observed that farms and stables that have a conscientious worm control program rarely have colic.

We are increasingly finding, though, that the effectiveness of the various drugs varies from ranch to ranch, and stable to stable. The only positive method of evaluating any worming method is to run microscopic studies of manure specimens (fecal examinations) before and after worming. All horse owners should do this occasionally to find out if their worming methods are really working. The specimens taken after the worming should be collected ten to fifteen days after the medication has been administered.

One of the saddest parts of associating with horses is that, if one is around them long enough, sooner or later one will see the heartbreaking death of a horse with colic. Even the mildest non-fatal colic is a pitiful sight to see. The agony of the affected horse is enough to make the stoniest heart weep. But most tragic of all is the fact that nearly all equine colics are preventable. So let's find out here and now how to prevent this malady and resolve to exercise every precaution so that our horses may be spared.

To begin with, the term colic is a vague one referring to any abdominal pain. Veterinarians speak of true colic and false colic. Depending on the severity of the pain, horses manifest colic by restlessness, stamping, stretching, straining, kicking or reaching with the nose at the abdomen, lying down, sweating, groaning, rolling, kicking backward, and finally, violent squealing and thrashing. False colic refers to pain arising from outside the digestive tract and includes such causes as kidney stones or infections, infections of the uterus, tumors, etc. True colic is pain arising from the digestive tract itself—that is, the stomach and intestine. In general, when we speak of colic we are referring to true colic.

The commonest causes of pain within the digestive tract of the horse are gas pressure, obstruction, spasms, inflammations, displacements of the organs, and obstruction of the arteries supplying the intestine.

As you can see, the complete diagnosis of colic involves, first, differing between false and true colic. Then, when true colic is established, it must be determined precisely where the pain is and what is causing it. The important thing for you, the horse owner, to understand is that true colic is usually the result of neglect, poor management, or feeding errors. Therefore, good management will produce a minimum of colic. I am going to list a long series of rules. Check them and see how many you break. Your horse may suffer and even die if you fail to observe these rules.

1/ Store feeds where it is impossible for horses to get at them accidentally. This is especially true of grains, green feeds, and new hay. Overeating such feeds causes very serious colics, often fatal.

2/ Never allow a horse access to spoiled food, such as moldy hay, filthy bedding, garbage, or stagnant water. Remember that the well-fed animal usually has little desire to eat unwholesome food. Break this rule and you risk forage poisonings and botulism as well as colic.

3/ Reduce the diet, especially grain,

when the horse is idle.

4/ Make any dietary changes gradually—such changes include the quantity, type, and quality of feeds. Sudden changes of feed invite colic.

5/ Do not feed on bare ground. Build a manger. Eating on the ground may produce sand colic, cause excessive wear of the teeth, and increase worminess due to the ingestion of manure containing worm eggs.

6/ Feed lightly when the horse is very tired. Fatigue often produces a reflex paralysis of the bowel. A similar effect can be produced by hunger or severe chilling.

7/ Don't feed or water, ever, when a horse is overheated.

8/ Check his teeth. Faulty teeth cause improper chewing, which in turn can result in colic.

9/ If you are graining heavily, split the ration between morning and evening. Graining *after* feeding hay is preferable to before.

10/ Feed at the same time, at least twice daily, at 12-hour intervals to prevent overloading of the digestive tract. Dividing the daily ration into three feedings, at approximately eight-hour intervals, is even better if this can be done.

11/ Keep him free from worms, particularly bloodworms. Otherwise, damaged arteries may plug with clots, causing thrombo-embolic colic.

12/ Feed decent hay. Avoid large quantities of finely chopped hays or, conversely, feeding coarse, heavy-stemmed roughage.

13/ Carrots or apples should be sliced.

14/ Ensure an abundant source of clean water. In very cold weather, horses may not consume enough water if the water is too cold.

15/ If colic should affect your horse, observe these first-aid measures until help arrives: Don't permit the animal to eat. Don't let him lie down or roll. Do trot him briskly around the corral.

Horses that die of colic usually succumb to a ruptured stomach or intestine, gangrene of the intestine, toxicity, or infection of the abdominal cavity. Like most diseases, colic is easier to prevent than it is to treat. Just remember that, with few exceptions, colic can be prevented.

SAND COLIC

As the popularity of pleasure horses increases, more people are keeping horses at their rural, suburban, and even city homes. Many of these horses are kept on rather small lots in densely populated subdivisions.

Some horse owners, who are rather inexperienced in the care and management of horses, wish to have an attractive corral, and want their horses in clean and comfortable surroundings. For these reasons, some owners will order a truckload of sand and carefully spread it around the corral.

Many horses kept in such sandy corrals have developed sand colic, or to use another common expression, they have become sanded. If your horse is being kept in such a corral, I hope that this article will awaken you to the potential danger that exists.

Veterinarians have always seen sanded horses, but for the reasons mentioned, this illness is becoming much more common. In our practice in southern California, we have had many families who, with all good intentions, dumped sand in their corrals. Ultimately, all of their horses developed sand colic and several horses died. In a couple of cases, we observed the sand long before the horses got sick and advised that it be removed. Regrettably, the owners did not heed our advice and, as predicted, these horses were eventually sanded.

When a horse eats sand, the heavier particles settle in the lower loops of the intestine. If a sufficient amount of sand accumulates, it irritates the bowel, causing pain, diarrhea, infection, and debility. A sudden heavy volume of sand ingested can completely block the digestive tract. Horses that die of sand colic might have 50 to 75 pounds of sand accumulated in their bowel. I once autopsied a horse with nearly 100 pounds of sand in his stomach, solidly packed into an impenetrable mass.

Horses eat sand for many reasons. First of all, the horse swallows a certain amount of sand when picking feed off the ground. But it takes a long time for the horse to accumulate enough sand in this manner to cause signs of discomfort because horses are remarkably adept at using their sensitive prehensile lips to pick up tiny bits of tasty feed, and avoiding anything undesirable.

Some horses develop a vice of eating soil. Such a depraved appetite is called *pica*. It is not unusual for a horse to eat a little soil. It is probably nature's way of supplying minerals. But if the soil contains a lot of heavy sand grains and the horse eats too much of it, he may get sand colic. Therefore, sand eating could theoretically result from a dietary deficiency.

For unknown reasons, some newborn foals will eat sand, and we have seen several cases of sand colic in baby foals. One foal, which had to be surgically saved, continued to crave sand and, even as a yearling, had to be muzzled except at feeding time.

Some horses will start to eat earth when they are sick, especially when they have a digestive upset. If there is a lot of sand in the soil, a simple case of indigestion could end up as a serious case of sand colic.

I once saw a shipment of alfalfa hay that had a spadeful of gravel and sand per flake. A horse could conceivably be sanded on such feed.

The horse with sand colic rarely displays severe pain. Usually the pain is moderate and intermittent. The horse often has diarrhea. The manure may have sand in it, but often the sand isn't obvious until after the horse is treated. Sometimes, upon rectal examination, the veterinarian can recover large handfuls of sand. In chronic sand colic, the horse is depressed, his mucus membranes become toxic looking, and he goes downhill rather rapidly.

We treat sanded horses by giving them large doses of mineral oil through a stomach tube, in the hope that this lubricant will help much of the sand to pass. Supportive treatment and pain-relieving drugs are also used. There is a human laxative product called Mucilose or Metamucil. It is a purified form of hemicellulose made from the seeds of the psyllium plant, and it comes in a dry, powdered form. Veterinary preparations of psyllium seed are now available. Once in the intestinal tract, Mucilose swells up tremendously, and as it passes through the bowel, it may pick up a lot of sand and facilitate its passage.

A pound of Mucilose may be given daily to the sanded horse. Some horses will eat the product dry, but more often the veterinarian will have to give it by stomach tube. Mucilose can quickly swell up and plug a stomach pump, so it is best sprinkled slowly into a gallon of mineral oil while an assistant vigorously pumps the oil through a tube into the horse.

COLIC SURGERY

If I were asked to name the single most dramatic advance in equine medicine since I entered the veterinary profession in 1956, it would have to be colic surgery. Colic is the most common cause of death in horses. The equine species, because of its anatomy, is particularly predisposed to obstruction of the digestive tract.

Now, I'm going to make a statement that may seem startling:

Most cases of colic can be saved.

Yes, most cases of colic that do not respond to simple conservative treatment can be saved if they are operated on. This is true today, but it wasn't true years ago. In fact, when I was a veterinary student, it was said, "If you open the belly of a horse, it will die." This wasn't invariably true. I can remember doing barnyard surgery on a few colics that did survive, but the majority of them did not. I used to wryly call such an operation an "ante-mortem post-mortem."

We are fortunate, in my area, to have several excellent equine hospitals available for us to refer major surgical cases to. They are not close. They are all 100 miles away, in various directions. It takes two hours to haul a colic case to a hospital, assuming that the owner of the horse has a trailer available. In spite of that, more than 90 percent of the colic cases we referred for surgery over a seven-year period returned home alive.

In our practice we see hundreds of colics annually. Our horse practice keeps four veterinarians busy. Most of these colics respond to conservative medical treatment. But, we refer about one case a week for surgery. A few of those recovered at the hospital without undergoing surgery. But the majority were operated and well over 90 percent were operated successfully.

Some of those cases would not be expected to recover. For example, in a two-year period, I can recall a 21-year-old mare that had to have 12 feet of bowel removed, an 18-year-old gelding that had 18 feet of intestine removed, and even a 25-year-old mare that was successfully operated.

We give credit for this phenomenal success rate to the hospital. They give the credit to us. We both must credit the owner. Let me explain:

1/ The owner must be willing to spend the money, and this decision must be made early. Colic surgery is expensive; the operation and aftercare will cost two, three, four thousand dollars. It is understandable when the owner says, "I just can't afford it, doctor. Do the best you can without operating." In spite of this, a majority of the horse owners in our practice today do go along with surgery.

There are more valuable horses around today—valuable monetarily and valued sentimentally. An increasing number of wise horse owners have surgical insurance on their horses. Also, more owners have witnessed abdominal surgery in the horse, and realize that the fees these equine hospitals charge are very low for what is done. Comparable procedures in the human, a much smaller and easier patient to operate, would be very much higher. It's time someone paid tribute to the increasing number of fine equine hospitals in this country and the superb job they do. Most of their operations are done at night, and the specialized equipment they use and the medications involved cost a fortune.

2/ The referring veterinarian must refer the case *early.* It is usually too late if one waits until the horse is dying. The attending veterinarian must make the difficult evaluation that this case is potentially surgical, and get the horse to an operating room in a fully equipped hospital (if one is available within a reasonable distance) without delay. The owner must help the veterinarian make that decision. Every horse owner should consider the possibility that his or her horse may someday require colic surgery, and decide now whether the answer is to be yes or no. Then, when a colic occurs, tell the veterinarian, "If surgery is required, I want you to know that I will go along with it. So, if there is that possibility, and a hospital is available, please don't hesitate to refer the case."

Again, the owner of a valued horse with foresight will have surgical insurance, or at least be prepared to stand the expense of surgery should the necessity arise.

3/ The hospital must have the surgical skill, the experience, the support staff, the monitoring equipment, the specialized anesthetic equipment, and material for supportive therapy if a high success rate is to be expected. Equine hospitals are, except for university teaching hospitals, privately financed. Their fees, as pointed out, are very low for what they do. Not every hospital can afford the requirements I listed above. An operating table is not all that is required. Many hospitals do the best they can with what they have, just as some small rural human hospitals have to get by as best they can. The kind of hospital I'm talking about costs hundreds of thousands of dollars, just to equip. The total investment may represent millions.

Many parts of the country have no such hospital. I practice in southern California where we have close to a million horses. We are fortunate, therefore, in having a number of good equine hospitals. In many other areas, there are *no* equine hospitals available, or perhaps a mortgaged veterinarian has equipped a facility as best he can. Most veterinarians are sincere and dedicated people who will do the best they can to save a horse. Their income comes from spending long hours doing routine things like worming, vaccinating, treating wounds, lameness, and respiratory infections. Major surgery is *not* profitable in the field of equine medicine. The establishment of an equine hospital requires sacrifice on the part of those who establish it.

I mentioned university hospitals. Let me add a comment. No university teaching hospital has a colic success rate of more than 90 percent. Most do well if they save half the patients they operate. The reason? Not because they lack the skill or the equipment. Hardly! In fact, most university teaching hospitals today have board-certified surgeons and the finest equipment. The problem, unfortunately, is that many of their patients are presented too late to be saved. Requirement number one, or two, or both were not fulfilled in time.

Yes, even university teaching hospital surgeons often do "ante-mortem post-mortems" as I did years ago, futilely operating on hopeless cases, already past the point of no return.

The success rate we have seen in our practice in referred colic surgery cases is wonderful. Rarely these days do we have to suffer what I used to call "the death watch"—attending a horse dying of colic. It was a frequent occurrence years ago in our practice, and it was horrible. It's still like that in many parts of our country, but year by year, the situation improves. New hospitals are established, and more horses are saved. Of course, nobody can guarantee that surgery will save a colic case. In a fragile species of such size and temperament, a lot of things can go wrong, but as the technology improves, fewer horses are lost to colic, and more survive.

Azoturia

Before the automobile age, azoturia was a common disease in work horses. In the light horses that prevail today, azoturia is not really common, but occurs often enough so that it behooves the average horseman to know a little about it. Azoturia is a disease in which certain muscles cramp and break down.

Old-timers may remember some of the old names for azoturia: Monday morning sickness, lumbago, and black water. Veterinarians also have synonyms for it. It is variously known as paralytic myoglobinuria, haemoglobinemia paralytica, or lumbar paralysis.

Azoturia attacks a horse suddenly. The muscles of any or all of the legs may be involved, but most often it is both hind legs that are affected, especially the massive muscles of the loin and hind-quarters. They become very hard, cramped, and painful if pressed. The horse's movements grow stiff and unco-ordinated. The muscles tremble. Due to pain, the horse sweats heavily. If he is moved, the condition rapidly worsens. If severe enough, the victim may sit down on his haunches like a dog, and finally he might go down and be unable to rise.

Due to the breakdown of muscle tissue, certain muscle pigments are released into the blood stream, which eventually find their way into the urine, causing it to become dark in color, sometimes as dark as black coffee. This is what gave rise to the name of black water disease. As the disease progresses, kidney function may fail completely. Most cases that go down, and are unable to rise, will eventually die. That is why it is so important that the horse be treated before he goes down.

There are two rules in azoturia: 1/ Don't move the horse, and 2/ Call a veterinarian as soon as possible.

Azoturia is a metabolic disease. This means that there is a disturbance in the chemistry of the body.

There is a certain history that is typical of azoturia. The horse is usually in good shape, on a high grain ration, and working hard every day. Then he is laid off for a day or two. When he goes back to work the attack starts, usually within 30 minutes of leaving the stall. You can see where the name of Monday morning sickness came from. Work horses in cities and on farms used to work very hard all week, and were grained heavily to keep them in good condition. Then, after having Sunday off, azoturia would strike when they were put back to work on Monday.

However, this typical history is by no means invariable. Azoturia might be seen in any horse, at any time, on any diet. For example, it might strike a horse that has been cast and tied down for shoeing or surgery, especially if no anesthetics or muscle relaxants were used. It may affect horses after long hauls in trailers or exhausting work. And, cases are sometimes seen in horses receiving no grain at all, and no exercise history typical of azoturia. Most cases, however, have the heavy grain and exercise routine preceding the attack.

It is interesting to note that azoturia is more common in the winter months, and most victims are young and fat. The mildest form of exercise precedes the attacks, sometimes after just a few minutes' work. One case I saw hit a mare after walking a few yards out of the stall.

Azoturia is often confused by the horseman with colic, founder, sleeping sickness, or kidney disease. The last is a favorite lay diagnosis. The urinary problems in azoturia are the *result* of the disease, not the *cause.* But countless gallons

It is interesting to note that azoturia is more common in the winter months, and most victims are young and fat.

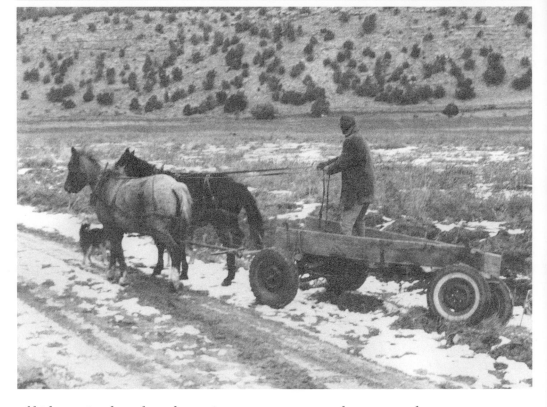

of kidney stimulants have been given to horses for centuries in the hope of preventing azoturia.

Most afflicted horses will recover, provided they don't go down. And, with modern drugs, even down cases can be saved.

Let's briefly discuss the treatment of azoturia. The most important immediate thing is *rest*. Avoid moving the horse. Feed no grain. The veterinarian has a variety of drugs useful in these cases, including thiamine to stimulate muscle metabolism, tranquilizers to relieve muscle spasm, cortisones to correct the severe inflammation and stress that occur, pain relievers, anti-inflammatory drugs, and alkalizers to neutralize the acid accumulations in muscle tissue. The use of preparations containing vitamin E and selenium are popular with equine practitioners treating muscle disorders. Very severe cases will require catheterization, intravenous fluid therapy, and possibly the use of muscle-relaxing drugs.

The greatest progress in handling azoturia has been the blood tests that measure certain enzymes that are liberated into the blood streams when muscle cells rupture. By means of these tests the veterinarian can confirm the diagnosis, tell how severe the attack is, know how long to treat the horse, and determine when recovery has occurred.

Once again, remember *not* to move the horse. I recall a case of a horse in Wyoming used to run down wild horses. One morning, after a day's rest, he was hit with severe azoturia five minutes out of camp. The owner led him back to camp, loaded the horse into a trailer, and rushed to the nearest veterinarian, some hours away. Moving the horse worsened the attack and the horse went down in the trailer. He died after three days of agony. I also recall several people who, thinking their horses had some sort of colic, forced them to *walk* with azoturia, thus worsening the case. If you think your horse has been attacked with azoturia, stop right there, leave the horse, and walk out for help.

Once a horse has had azoturia, he will be predisposed to further attacks. Feed such a horse lightly on grain, and exercise him daily.

Azoturia, like so many diseases, can usually be prevented with proper management. Don't overwork any horse, especially if he is out of shape. Don't grain too heavily if he is idle. Ask your veterinarian if you are in a selenium-deficient area. Before shipping fat horses long distances, it might be wise to tranquilize them. If a well-conditioned horse in hard physical condition must be laid off, especially in a confined space, cut his grain ration drastically, and give a bran mash the first day to flush his digestive tract.

I'd like to say a word now about *tying-up* in race horses, also known as *cording-up* or myositis. Authorities differ as to whether this is the same as azoturia. There are many similarities. For example, the symptoms of a tied-up horse resemble a mild case of azoturia. Certain enzyme tests on the blood serum show the same changes in both conditions.

On the other hand, there are differences. Tying-up is more common in mares. We don't see the kidney damage in tying-up that we do in azoturia. Azoturia usually shows the work-grain-rest history, whereas tying-up occurs during training, in animals working hard every day. Possibly tying-up is a form of azoturia that is aborted because the horse is usually rested as soon as it appears. Some tied-up horses, however, seem to improve if exercised. That is, the muscle spasm "works itself out." It is likely that two separate conditions affect the race horse, both labelled tying-up: 1/ true azoturia, and 2/ muscle cramping and spasm due to overwork.

Considerable research is being done both here and abroad to help us understand these ancient muscle diseases.

Equine Rhinopneumonitis

Equine rhinopneumonitis is a common virus disease of horses caused by a DNA virus called *Equine herpesvirus one*, or EHV/1. It is an upper respiratory infection and resembles a human cold. Although young horses are more susceptible, horses of any age can contract this disease.

The name rhinopneumonitis means inflammation of the nose and lungs, and symptoms include coughing, nasal discharge, and sometimes swollen glands. Some cases run a fever and are quite sick. Other cases are affected to a lesser degree and just seem to have a mild cold. Of course, "rhino," as most horsemen refer to it, is contagious and epidemics are common on farms and in stables.

When a susceptible horse is exposed to the virus, it will usually incubate seven to ten days before causing visible symptoms. Most cases last a week or two before recovering. It is important that sick horses not be exercised, and that they have good nursing care. The more severely affected cases, especially those with signs of secondary bacterial infection (fever, swollen glands, thick nasal discharge), should be seen by a veterinarian.

Doesn't sound too serious, does it? Kind of like a bad cold, right? Wrong! This is a *very* serious disease that formerly caused devastating losses in our horse industry every year. The rhino virus can cause abortion in pregnant mares. This is the same virus that causes equine viral abortion. When the virus grows in the pregnant mare's blood stream, a "viremia," or infection of the blood stream, occurs, that spreads to the fetus. The mare will then abort a few weeks to several months later. Or, the mare might carry the foal to full term, but it will be born weak and will die after birth.

The rhino virus occurs all over the world, and in this country it causes many more abortions in some areas than it does in others. The more horses in a given area, the more favorable are conditions for a serious outbreak. Horses traveling between shows, racetracks, and farms keep spreading the virus. And the stress of traveling, weaning, or inclement weather increases the susceptibility to rhino. The presence of young, non-immune foals and immature horses also makes outbreaks more likely.

A less common form of the disease is the neurological form. In this devastating variation, the virus attacks the brain, and usually the horse will eventually die. The neurological form of rhino might occur alone, or in combination with the respiratory and/or abortion form.

The virus does produce immunity in an exposed horse, but unfortunately, the immunity is of rather short duration. A horse can have this disease year after year.

Foals are born with no protection against the virus, but if the dam is immune, she will pass temporary protecting antibodies to the foal through her first milk, or colostrum. However, this immunity wears off in a few weeks, so it is important to immunize suckling foals early.

One of the first immunization methods to protect against rhino was unusual. A technique was developed for giving a band of horses the actual disease at a favorable time when no pregnant mares could abort. The virus was sprayed into the horses' noses while they underwent a quarantine period. After they recovered from the disease, mares were bred. They had temporary immunity and they could, hopefully, carry their foals to term without virus abortion occurring.

This method of controlled infection was far from ideal, but it did help to prevent costly "abortion storms" on breeding farms.

Finally, true vaccines were developed. There are two kinds of vaccine: modified live virus and killed virus. Both vaccines are safe and effective, and thanks to them, losses of fetuses from this virus have become relatively uncommon.

The respiratory and neurological forms of this disease are still with us, however. The incidence of their occurring can be greatly diminished by boostering all immunized horses frequently— at least every six months, and even more often for horses frequently exposed.

In our practice, we adopted a method of protecting mares and foals against equine rhinopneumonitis that was developed by Dr. D.M. Witherspoon, the veterinarian for Spendthrift Farm in Lexington, Ky., a leading Thoroughbred farm.

Foals are inoculated with the modified live virus vaccine at 30, 60, and 90 days of age. Then they are boostered every two months until May of their yearling year. Broodmares are immunized every 30 days.

With this method, Dr. Witherspoon found that the incidence of the disease on Spendthrift Farm was controlled. The breeding farms in our own practice that have used this method have had similar good results, and there have been no adverse effects from the frequent use of the vaccine.

The incidence of complicating foal pneumonia has also been greatly reduced, and virus abortion in mares does not occur.

Tetanus

Tetanus, once known as lockjaw, is a disease of special interest to the horseman for two reasons: First, the germ that causes tetanus—*Clostridium tetani*—is a common inhabitant in horse manure. Secondly, horses are more susceptible to the infection than other animals. For example, a dog is 300 times more resistant to tetanus toxin than a horse. So, you can see that since horses are so sensitive to this disease, and actually carry the causative bacteria in their own intestine, it behooves every horseman to thoroughly understand this terrible illness.

The tetanus germ doesn't mean to hurt anybody. You see, he's ordinarily a harmless fellow who likes to live in soil and in manure. He reproduces by forming spores. Now these spores will not "hatch" in the presence of oxygen. They will only grow in airless places such as deep in the soil, or in deep wounds, such as created by a sliver, an insect bite, or a nail puncture.

As the bacterial colony grows, it throws off waste products, as do all living things. One of these waste products, by sheer coincidence, happens to be a deadly poison. This poison, known as *tetanus toxin,* attacks the nerves of the victim, causing the spasms and rigid paralysis that is typical of the disease. The horse, cow, sheep, dog, human, or other unfortunate creature with tetanus suffers horrible paralytic spasms of the jaw muscles (hence "lockjaw") and other muscles of the body. In an advanced case the entire victim may be as rigid as a statue. After prolonged suffering, the majority of such patients die.

The death nowadays of either a horse or a human being from tetanus is an inexcusable case of negligence.

Every horse and every person, whether or not he works around horses, should be immunized against tetanus!

Immunization against tetanus is accomplished with the use of tetanus toxoid. What is toxoid? It is a harmless and deactivated tetanus toxin. Two injections are given, 30 to 60 days apart. Thereafter, in horses, a once-a-year booster is all that is necessary to keep immunity at a high level. If you neglect the boosters, and a wound occurs, an immediate restoration of immunity will occur if a toxoid booster is given at once, even if it has been many years since the original injections were given. However, it is better to give a booster every year instead of waiting for a wound to occur. Why? Because many tetanus-causing wounds in horses are never seen by the owner. For example, consider splinters, barbed wire punctures, and being "quicked" by a horseshoe nail. One point must be made clear. The first two tetanus toxoid injections should be given *before* an injury occurs.

Now, what if your horse has never been immunized—has never had tetanus toxoid, and he suffers a wound? How can you protect him against tetanus? Well, in a case of this kind we use tetanus antitoxin. Please get this straight. Antitoxin is different from toxoid. It does *not* permanently protect against tetanus, but only for about two weeks.

Obviously, it is much better to rely on active immunity with tetanus toxoid than it is to rely on passive immunity with tetanus antitoxin. But, the veterinarian will use antitoxin in case of a wound or a surgical operation, unless you tell him that the horse has been previously immunized with toxoid.

The use of tetanus toxoid is a very safe procedure in horses and in people. Millions of servicemen, and nearly all babies, now receive toxoid. New vaccines are available that combine tetanus toxoid with several other vaccines.

Suppose you have been careless, and your horse contracts tetanus. Is there a cure? No, there isn't a specific cure. But much can be done to help the patient. Doctors treat tetanus by cleaning up the causative wound, using antibiotics and large amounts of antitoxin to prevent further damage, force-feeding to keep strength up, and other supportive therapy. Some of the new muscle-relaxing and tranquilizing drugs have been of great value.

But, despite all efforts, most horses with tetanus continue to die, as do an unfortunate number of human patients.

Please note that in many cases of tetanus, there is no obvious wound. For this reason alone every horse and every person should be protected against tetanus, with tetanus toxoid. Do not wait until a wound occurs to consult your physician and your veterinarian.

Tetanus toxoid is remarkably effective, and so easily administered. A death from tetanus is an unnecessary tragedy in a disease so easily prevented.

Remember the following: 1/ Horses are far more susceptible than humans to develop tetanus; 2/ Most tetanus victims die; 3/ The tetanus germ is commonly found in manure and barnyard soil; and 4/ The tetanus germ cannot grow in the presence of oxygen, so deep wounds—particularly punctures—are the most dangerous.

Equine Influenza ("Flu")

Those of us with horses who experienced the 1963 epidemic of equine flu will not soon forget it. The flu first appeared in Florida, during the month of February, in some Thoroughbreds flown in from South America. In a few weeks the disease spread like wildfire on the Florida racetracks and then fanned out across the country. By June, the epidemic had spread to all parts of the country, causing great problems at race meets and horse shows.

The virus was eventually identified as a new strain, and named A-2-Equine Influenza Virus, and it will probably be with us permanently.

Equine influenza is similar to human flu. There are many strains of flu virus. During most years the disease is mild, but once in a while severe epidemics or worldwide *pandemics* occur with devastating results. Human flu vaccines have been available for many years. Horses can also be vaccinated against influenza. Influenza usually appears in the spring. There are government-approved vaccines available for immunizing horses against flu. The vaccines contain two strains of equine flu virus.

Diagnosing influenza is difficult, even for a veterinarian. Flu resembles other respiratory diseases of horses, such as viral arteritis, distemper, and rhinopneumonitis. All of these diseases involve fever, coughing, and nasal discharge. Accurate differentiation requires laboratory tests. Moreover, the influenza virus cannot be destroyed by using antibiotics in horses (or in humans). Antibiotics are only of use to control secondary bacterial complications. Obviously, prevention is much simpler than a cure, and that's why I advise that all horses be vaccinated against flu.

Since the 1963 epidemic, equine flu has occurred sporadically. However, history assures us that, sooner or later, another explosion will occur. During World War I, thousands of Army horses died of influenza. An epidemic struck Sweden and eastern Europe in 1956 and central Europe in 1979. The 1963 American epidemic certainly won't be our last.

Horsemen must realize that the equine flu vaccines now available offer an immunity of short duration. They must be boostered periodically, as recommended by your local veterinarian.

Heaves

The horse with true heaves has it for life. Horses that are said to have been cured of heaves probably had chronic bronchitis rather than heaves.

Heaves in horses is often called *broken wind.* This term is somewhat misleading. For example, a *roarer* may be called broken-winded. Yet roaring is caused by a paralyzed membrane in the larynx, up in the throat. True heaves, on the other hand, is a disease of the lungs.

Veterinarians know heaves as chronic *pulmonary alveolar emphysema,* and these medical terms accurately describe the disease. It *is* chronic. The horse with true heaves has it for life. Horses that are said to have been cured of heaves probably had chronic bronchitis rather than heaves.

To describe heaves, we must explain that the pulmonary alveoli are the millions of tiny air sacs in the lungs. They give the lungs their spongy quality. In heaves, these sacs lose their elasticity. They rupture and break down to form spaces filled with residual air. This condition we call *emphysema.* Thus heaves is chronic *pulmonary alveolar emphysema.*

Heaves is not often seen in young horses. Most horses with heaves are at least five years old. However, an occasional case may follow a respiratory infection in younger horses. Also, horses that are suddenly transported from very high altitude to sea level may be predisposed to this disease.

A cough is the first noticeable symptom of heaves. The owner will assume it is an ordinary cough due to a cold or dust. But this cough hangs on. It becomes worse when the horse is exercised or exposed to dust. The cough might be quite mild, but occasional severe paroxysms might alarm the owner. Such a severe attack will usually occur after exercise, feeding, drinking cold water, or coming out of a warm barn into cold air.

At this point the veterinarian, listening with a stethoscope, can detect the characteristic wheezing lung sounds of early heaves. As time goes on, other symptoms develop. If you put your ear to the horse's chest, you can easily hear the long, drawn-out wheezing sound. Since the lungs have lost their normal elasticity, the horse has to force the air out of them when he breathes out. In order to do this, he will contract the abdominal muscles at the end of each breath. Thus he breathes *in* normally, but breathes *out* with two distinct movements. If a mirror is held in front of a nostril, the double expiration can be seen clearly.

Horses that have heaves a long time develop big barrel chests. The ribs are sprung far apart. The diaphragmatic muscles enlarge. A pot belly develops from the stretched abdominal muscles. A furrow at the muscle attachments develops along the ribs, extending up toward the hip. This furrow is called the "heave line."

The heart gradually enlarges and is weakened. The horse is short-winded and has no stamina. He can become unthrifty and remain in poor condition. Some cases have a nasal discharge.

Due to the labored breathing, the horse tends to swallow a lot of air. This causes flatulence. He will pass a lot of odorous gas. There may be chronic indigestion and diarrhea. The food is poorly digested. Eventually this can cause anemia and malnutrition.

If the heart weakness is severe enough, edema will develop. This means that fluid accumulated in the lower part of the body causes the legs, or even the lower abdomen, to swell. Naturally, dust and exercise worsen the symptoms and tend to bring on severe attacks. Some chronic cases of heaves show a depraved appetite. Such a horse may eat dirt or manure.

The cause of heaves is debatable. The two things considered most likely are infection and allergy. It is possible that, as in human asthma, both factors play a role in causing the disease. And, again, as in human asthma, there may be other factors we do not yet fully understand.

Some cases certainly seem to follow a respiratory infection that causes a chronic bronchitis. But the most generally accepted theory is that the horse is allergic to some substance he inhales.

We know that most cases are aggravated by feeding legume hays such as alfalfa or clover, especially if it is dusty or moldy. Perhaps legume hays are more prone to mold growth; and it is the mold spores that the horse inhales that precipitate the attack.

The symptoms of heaves can be masked for several hours by giving the horse an injection of atropine. This trick has long been used by unscrupulous horse traders. You can tell if a horse has had atropine by his dry mouth and dilated pupils of the eyes. Fasting the horse is another trick to conceal heaves—not allowing food or water for at least 12 hours. With the stomach empty, the lungs expand more easily, and the heaves might not be readily noticeable. Naturally, the best way to avoid buying a horse that might have heaves is to have a licensed veterinarian give the horse a thorough and competent examination.

Heaves is a progressive disease. With each attack more alveoli are permanently worn down, and the emphysema grows increasingly worse. So although there is no *cure* for heaves, it is important to *control* the disease.

A lot can be done in the way of control. The lungs must not be strained by exhausting running, pulling heavy loads, or roping and dragging heavy cattle. Do not feed legume hay. (To avoid misunderstanding, let me hasten to say that legume hay is an excellent feed for horses that don't have heaves.) Instead, feed small amounts of the best quality native meadow grass hay or prairie hay. If possible, cut the hay and sprinkle it with water, or better still, sprinkle it with lime water. If you can't get such hay, use timothy hay, but it is not as good as prairie hay.

Better yet, put the horse on green pasture. A horse with heaves might remain free of symptoms on pasture.

Feed the horse plenty of whole oats to reduce the amount of hay necessary. A little corn is good, too. Be sure all feed is free of dust. If it isn't, sprinkle it with water.

Complete pelleted rations are a good way to feed a horse with heaves. Pelleted feeds are less dusty than hay, and the pelleting process causes heat that destroys mold spores. Many horses with heaves improve when they are fed only pelleted feed. Beet pulp is also a good roughage. Sliced carrots are beneficial. A vitamin-mineral supplement is indicated, but I would avoid the powdered kind. Instead, use a pellet, granule, liquid, or candied type.

Water the horse before feeding instead of after. Never work a horse with heaves on a full stomach. Keep him from both feed and water for a few hours before working him.

There are several drugs that offer relief to horses suffering from heaves. They include antihistamines, cortisones, and bronchodilators. Your veterinarian can prescribe commercial products containing stramonium that are beneficial. A compound containing belladona in Fowler's solution was popular years ago. Acupuncture has been reported to relieve heaves.

There might be an inheritable predisposition to heaves, so serious consideration to this possibility should be given before breeding a horse suffering from this disease.

If heaves is an uncomplicated allergic disease, the horse owner can't do much in the way of preventive medicine for the horse. However, certain fundamental rules of good horse care should be observed. For example, if the hay or corral is dusty, sprinkle with water.

If your horse ever develops a cough, *stop* all exercise until the cough is gone. If it is severe or persistent, consult a veterinarian about a diagnosis and medication.

Equine Infectious Anemia

Equine Infectious Anemia, also known as swamp fever, is a communicable virus disease of horses and other equine-type animals. It occurs in many parts of the world including the United States. The disease is serious, not so much because of its prevalence, but because there is no treatment that is effective against this virus, nor is there a vaccine yet known capable of immunizing a horse against the disease. Occasional outbreaks at racetracks, farms, or stables present a very serious problem.

EIA occurs widely all over the United States, but we now have a test, the Coggins test, that can reliably detect the disease, including the carrier state. Coggins tests are required by many states prior to allowing horses into the state, and are also frequently required by sales, shows, and fairs.

Many horses with EIA die. Others survive the disease, and these survivors can act as carriers, serving as a source of infection for other horses. The virus may be carried from the blood stream of a carrier to the blood stream of a susceptible horse by biting insects, or by nonsterile hypodermic needles.

Once the virus enters the body, it attacks many organs, causing a variety of symptoms. Some cases are mild and some fatally severe. Some cases are acute, and others chronic, running a prolonged course before terminating in either death or recovery. Acute cases may display fever, sweating, and great depression. Such cases may die very quickly or the disease may taper off to take on a chronic form.

Chronic cases of swamp fever are more common. Such horses show a fluctuating low fever, anemia, loss of weight, increasing weakness, poor appetite, jaundice, staggering or paralysis, hemorrhages of the mucus membranes, and frequent urination.

Since there is neither a specific cure for the disease nor a preventive vaccine, our main line of defense against it is accurate diagnosis. The veterinarian attending the case will send a blood sample from the patient to a laboratory for special tests. Confirmed cases must be removed so that they cannot serve as a source of infection for other horses.

Hypodermic needles, syringes, surgical instruments, and tattooing instruments used on horses must always be sterilized for each animal.

Skin Diseases

Dermatology is one of the most complex branches of medical science. There-fore we will not try to cover *all* of the many skin diseases that can afflict the horse. Instead, we will consider just a few of the more common skin lesions seen in horses in the United States.

Warts (Papillomatosis) are found quite often in young horses. They appear as scattered nodules on the lips and nose or elsewhere. Horsemen often call them blood warts or seed warts. In severe cases there may be hundreds of small individual warts on the muzzle. Warts are caused by a virus and are spread from one animal to another by infected fences, curry combs, and other equipment around the stable. If left alone, these warts will usually disappear in two or three months. If for any reason they need to be removed more quickly, they may be taken off surgically. Castor oil applied to the warts might hasten their disappearance. If warts are a real problem in a stable, a special vaccine may be prepared to immunize young stock against the disease. Cattle wart vaccines are not effective in treating warts in the horse.

Horses sometimes get a flat, dry persistent type of wart inside the ear. These may be treated with castor oil. Occasional severe cases respond to X-ray therapy.

Remember that the ordinary little warts seen so often on the muzzle of young horses will nearly always disappear without treatment.

Allergic dermatitis: Many horses suffer from an itchy rash every summer. The lesions, in a typical case, are found mostly on the neck, face, shoulders, chest, and front legs. Or, the mane and base of the tail may be involved. Sometimes they occur on the hind legs, too. During the winter the inflammation clears up and the hair grows back until the skin is virtually normal. But when summer returns, the lesions return.

Allergic dermatitis occurs in horses all over the world. It is often called summer itch, summer eczema, or fungus itch. In Arizona we called it caliche itch or adobe itch, and in California it is Spanish itch or California itch. In Australia a similar condition is known as Queensland itch, and I'm sure dozens of other names are used wherever horses are found.

Allergic dermatitis may be caused by

an allergy to almost any substance. The higher incidence during the summer has cast suspicion on green pastures, pollens, heat, and excessive sweating. I personally believe that the majority of horses with allergic dermatitis are hypersensitive to biting flies. It is interesting to note that summer eczema in dogs, which was blamed on diet, heat, fungus, and everything else, is now recognized by authorities to be a simple allergic dermatitis caused, in a majority of cases, by hypersensitivity to the bite of the common flea.

Similarly, some horses are especially sensitive to biting flies, and I think that flies account for most cases of summer itch in horses.

There are many old-time treatments for allergic dermatitis, but none of them are as effective as the newer antihistamines and other anti-allergic drugs. These drugs offer prompt and lasting relief. Medicated baths and washes help to speed recovery. Obviously, a good fly control program, sanitation, and the use of fly repellent sprays on the horse himself every morning will all help to relieve summer itch. Keeping the horse in a cool, fly-free barn will help most cases.

Hives (Urticaria), also known as nettlerash or surfeit, also is an allergic reaction—most often to some substance in the diet. The horse is covered with flat-topped swellings. In severe cases the face is swollen, especially the eyelids and nose. Severe swelling of the nose can be dangerous since it interferes with breathing. Hives are quite common in horses; for some reason, however, the owner is usually surprised to learn this. Hives respond miraculously to injections of antihistamine or cortisone. A laxative is indicated if the sensitizing substance is in the digestive tract.

Photosensitization is the last type of skin allergy we will describe. It is caused by sensitization to sunlight and is therefore most often seen in the sunny western states. Don't confuse photosensitization with sunburn. We are discussing a severe *allergic* reaction to sunlight. The parts of the skin involved are white or unpigmented. Thus a sorrel or bay horse may only have lesions on a white-stockinged foot, or a bald-faced horse may have only the white part of his face affected. The unpigmented nose and lips

are common sites. Paint horses may have all of the white parts of their body damaged, while the dark areas remain normal. The skin lesions start with redness and inflammation, resembling a burn. Then serum oozes from the skin. Later the lesions peel. In severe cases the skin dies completely and sloughs away.

What causes photosensitization? Why doesn't *every* horse with white skin develop the disease? Well, there are several causes of photosensitization. Certain plants, such as buckwheat and St. John's wart, may contain toxic substances that sensitize skin unprotected by pigment to sunlight. Certain chemicals, including the bloodworm remedy phenothiazine, can occasionally cause similar sensitization. Rarely, an inherited allergy to sunlight occurs.

Lastly, a great variety of plants can sometimes damage the liver, causing chemical changes in the body leading to sunlight sensitivity. Such plants include clover, vetch, puncture vine, agave, lantana, alfalfa, lucerne, and others. Sometimes the disease is named after the Latin name of the plant involved. Thus photosensitization caused by eating toxic clover may be called *Trifoliosis;* or that caused by eating puncture vine (Tribulis terrestris) may be described as *Tribulosis.*

The treatment, obviously, involves first removing the horse from sunlight. A dark stall is ideal. Next, the causative agents must be identified, and removed. If it is a plant, which is usually the case, that plant must not be fed to the horse. Again, injections of antihistamines and cortisone preparations are very effective in relieving the symptoms and promoting recovery.

Ringworm is one of the most frequently seen skin diseases in horses. It is caused by a variety of fungi that attack the hair and skin, and sometimes the hoofs of the horse. Fungi are plants. Some are large and include the mushroom family. Other fungi are microscopic in size, and some of them cause diseases in animals and people. The term ringworm has nothing to do with worms, and the skin lesions do not always have circular or ring-like form, so it confuses many people. For example, I often find that riders think that their horse cannot catch ringworm if they have their horse wormed.

True ringworm is contagious. Some kinds of ringworm are communicable to dogs, cats, and other animals as well as to humans.

Ringworm in horses is also known as girth itch, fungus itch, and Spanish itch; and there are many other colloquial names for these fungus infections.

Since there are many different kinds of skin fungi that cause ringworm, the appearance of the disease is very variable. It may show as one or more scaly hairless spots anywhere on the body. Or there may be large hairless areas. Sometimes the lesions are thick and crusty, and ooze. Some are raw, and some are not. Some kinds of ringworm itch, but most do not. Even a veterinarian can never say for sure without laboratory tests if a skin disease is ringworm caused by a fungus, or if it's some other kind of dermatitis. Horses get many kinds of skin disease, and a specific diagnosis is sometimes difficult to achieve. This is true of skin diseases in people, pet animals, and in livestock as well as it is in horses.

Ringworm fungi produce spores. When these microscopic spores contact the skin of a susceptible horse, they grow into a fungus that grows on the hair and upper skin surface, attacking it, and killing the hair.

It is said that ringworm can be contracted by airborne spores, but I don't believe that a normal individual will get the disease unless the spores are rubbed into the skin. Thus, stiff-bristled grooming brushes, curry combs, electric clippers, cinches, halters, and saddle blankets usually carry the infection from one animal to another. For this reason, I see most cases at stables where the horses get lots of grooming and good care. Ringworm is seen less often in pastured horses that are seldom groomed.

Laboratory tests are necessary to positively identify ringworm, although experienced veterinarians can often guess the diagnosis from the appearance of the lesions.

Ringworm is usually not a serious disease, although it will often cause panic in a stable. For this reason, I usually call it a fungus infection (which it is). This doesn't excite anyone; whereas if I call it ringworm, people start pulling their horses out of the stable and transferring them to other stables (which might also have ringworm). Some people react to the term ringworm as they would to the word leprosy. In each case, overreaction is unjustified.

Most cases of ringworm will get well if just left alone. However, we don't recommend this because healing can be greatly accelerated with treatment, and also because once in a while a case will become chronic and generalized, and refuse to get well. Some patients develop lifetime infections of the hair or hoof.

The treatment of ringworm takes a little time, but is simple. The spots must be treated with something that kills the fungus.

There are dozens of treatments available that are effective in the treatment of ringworm. Your veterinarian probably has several favorites. Too-frequent treatment, or too many medicines, can irritate the skin and cause as much trouble as the fungus itself.

In addition to topical treatment (application of fungicidal medicine to the actual infected area), it is helpful to wash the entire body with a fungicidal shampoo (many brands are available, most containing either tamed povidol iodine or a sulphur compound), or with a fungicidal dip.

In stubborn cases, Griseofulvin, an oral antibiotic, may be prescribed. This can be fed daily mixed with the feed or a large dose can be administered all at one time through a stomach tube, and repeated in ten days.

The affected horse should not be groomed with a comb or brush until well. Don't use the affected horse's tack on other horses. Disinfect equipment in one of the fungicidal dips or you can use ordinary household chlorine bleach, diluted with water to disinfectant strength. See the label. Soak curry combs, brushes, etc., in the disinfectant overnight.

Ringworm can be prevented by not swapping equipment or tack, by disinfecting clipper blades after every use, and by early recognition and prompt isolation of the infected horse.

Summer sores (Cutaneous habronemiasis) is a stubborn skin problem in horses. Most horsemen know it as summer sores, but the disease has also been called bursatti, boil, dermatitis granulosa, and jack sores. The last name originated because of the prevalence of these sores on donkeys and mules.

These nasty sores are found most often on the legs, flanks, back, neck, and penis of the horse. They start as inflamed lesions that refuse to heal. Soon, ulcerations and rawness appear. The sore grows—sometimes reaching massive proportions. These sores resemble proud flesh.

Summer sores are caused by the migrating larvae of common stomach worms of the horse (habronema and draschia). The worm eggs pass out in the manure. Then fly maggots eat the eggs. The adult fly deposits the eggs on wounds accidentally when feeding on the wound. The eggs hatch, and the larvae migrate into the tissues, causing great irritation.

Summer sores are most common in warm climates. The susceptibility to such lesions seems to vary from one horse to another. During the winter the sores tend to heal spontaneously, only to break out again next summer.

Because summer sores resemble simple proud flesh, benign tumors, and cancer, an accurate diagnosis is necessary. Microscopic examination and scrapings taken from the sore will reveal the worm larvae if there is any question as to the diagnosis.

Treating summer sores is not easy. A great variety of treatments have been used, mostly with limited success.

Ointments containing cortisone and antibiotics suppress much of the inflammation and rawness in the sore, but they have no effect on the larvae. Old, chronic sores are often best treated by removing them surgically. The worming drug Ivermectin is effective in controlling migrating habronema larvae, and should be part of the treatment. Some veterinarians use compounds containing insecticides and other ingredients in a DMSO base to treat summer sores.

To prevent this problem, keep horses wormed, keep flies under control, and protect all wounds from flies. Use a fly-repellent dressing if necessary.

Eye Problems

The eye is a unique organ. The eye is a complicated structure, delicate and fragile in some ways, and amazingly tough in others. A neglected minor infection, or a blow, can sometimes lead to permanent blindness. Yet, the eye surgeon boldly opens the eyeball and works inside it successfully. Generally speaking, horses don't have a lot of eye trouble. There are, however, a few conditions that seem to be fairly prevalent.

Injury— to the eyeball or the surrounding structures is the most common eye problem. Barbed wire, tree limbs, and kicks by another horse frequently lacerate and bruise the eyelids, conjunctival membranes, or the eyeball itself. Careful surgical repair of the surrounding structures is important to prevent disfigurement. The eyeball itself should be promptly and skillfully treated to relieve pain, prevent infection, and encourage healing.

The eyeball that has been injured will often turn blue or milky in color. This doesn't mean that the horse will necessarily remain blind, and this opacity of the cornea (outer skin of the eyeball) is not a cataract. A cataract is an opacity of the lens, deep inside the eye. (Opacity is the state of a body that makes it impervious to light rays.) The blue or milky eye I described is often mistakenly called a cataract by the horse owner. With time and proper medication this opacity can usually be cleared up. If it is neglected, infection of the cornea and inflammation of the interior of the eyeball can follow.

Infection—When the cornea is damaged, and the injury is neglected, infection nearly always will follow. This is the reason that even a minor eye injury should receive scrupulous attention. An infected cornea may ulcerate. An ulcerated cornea may perforate. A perforated cornea may terminate in blindness. Many horses have been blinded by relatively minor eye problems that were neglected.

Infections of the eye can be due to other things. For example, foals with strangles (distemper) sometimes develop *hypopyon*, which is an accumulation of pus inside the eyeball. In hypopyon, you can actually see the pus inside the eye by looking through the transparent cornea.

Flies are a common cause of conjunctivitis or pinkeye. Flies love to gather

Many horses have been blinded by relatively minor eye problems that were neglected.

65

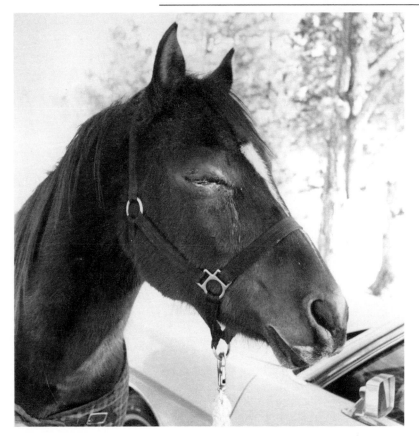

around the horse's eyes. They irritate the eyes and infection follows. Such eyes run tears and pus, have red membranes, and in severe cases may show considerable swelling of the lids. An antibiotic will clear up the infection, and you can prevent its recurrence by using a fly repellent *around* the eye. Never apply repellent above the eye, for if it rains, the repellent will then wash into the eye. Ask your veterinarian to suggest a safe brand of repellent.

Flies are also responsible for "summer sores," or *habronemiasis*, involving the inner corner of the eyelids. The flies carry the eggs of a worm, habronema, and they hatch. The microscopic habronema larvae, migrating through the tissues, cause summer sores. The worming drug Ivermectin is effective against habronema, but local treatment by a veterinarian is also indicated.

Sometimes, foreign material such as mud or the foxtail awns of wild oats or barley seeds will work under the eyelids and cause infection. There is also a small parasite called an eye worm *(Thelazia lacrimalis* or *Thelazia californensis)* that occasionally invades the eyes of the horse, although it is more common in cattle and dogs. This worm will also

cause infection.

Infected eyes often lead to infected tear ducts. The tears of a horse, like our own, drain through a little hole in the inner corner of the eyelid, and then through the lacrimal canal, into the nose. If the duct becomes plugged with infected matter, the tears have no place to go except to run down the face. The veterinarian flushes the plugged tear duct from the nose end, rather than from the eye.

Cancer of the eyelids, especially in pinto, Appaloosa, or white horses, is not at all unusual, and we cover this topic in detail in another chapter on cancer.

Periodic ophthalmia— Certainly no discussion of equine eye diseases is complete without mentioning this very serious ailment. Periodic ophthalmia is also called *recurrent iridocyclitis* or *uveitis.* In the old days it was known as moon blindness because horsemen mistakenly thought the disease was related to the phases of the moon.

This disease is the most common reason for blindness in the horse. The cause has been attributed to many things other than the moon. A few years back it was blamed on a riboflavin (a B vitamin) deficiency. Streptococcal infections (such as strangles) and parasitic larvae have also been incriminated. Another theory is that periodic ophthalmia is related to leptospirosis infection. The leptospira are a family of corkscrew-shaped bacteria that cause infections in many species. There is some scientific evidence at this time to support the theory that leptospirosis can cause periodic ophthalmia. Apparently, periodic ophthalmia can be caused by many things, including parasite migration and an allergic-type reaction in the horse's tissue.

The horse with periodic ophthalmia initially shows inflammation of one or both eyes. The pupil is contracted, the eye is sensitive to light, and excessive tears may stream down the face. These attacks last for indefinite periods and recur from time to time. Each attack damages the eye until, ultimately, the horse goes blind.

There is no cure for periodic ophthalmia, but the attack can be treated effectively, the horse relieved of his pain, and blindness postponed. It is very important that the veterinarian be called as soon as possible after the attack begins, because the longer the attack is allowed to last without treatment, the greater the permanent damage done to the eye. There is no reliable method of preventing the attacks. The feeding of riboflavin is of questionable value, but certainly can do no harm and is therefore advised.

Horses have many more eye problems than those we have covered. They include cataracts, dislocated lens, congenital malformations, and a variety of diseases of the retina and other structures within the eye. But these have no place in the horseman's manual because they are treated rarely, even by veterinarians.

When horsemen speak of a glass-eyed horse, they refer to an eye that is any color other than normal, but the eye is usually some shade of blue. A *china eye* is blue, a *wall eye* is part blue and part white, and a *watch eye* is a mixture of yellow and blue.

Glass eyes are hereditary, and may be seen in any kind of horse, although they are most common in Appaloosas and paints. A horse may have two glass eyes, or one glass eye and one normal eye. Horses with glass eyes have perfectly normal vision. There are a lot of old wives' tales around about such horses having poor vision or being susceptible to snow blindness. A glass-eyed horse is no more susceptible to snow blindness than a blue-eyed man as compared to a brown-eyed man. One often hears that glass-eyed horses are night-blind. This is not ordinarily true.

However, some glass-eyed horses lack a *tapetum lucidum.* This is a patch of pigmented tissue at the back of the eyeball. The tapetum lucidum reflects light and improves night vision. It is the tapetum lucidum that causes the eyes of the animal to glow in the dark.

Glass-eyed horses that tend toward albinoism may lack the tapetum lucidum, and therefore cannot see as well at night as most horses do.

Another popular fallacy is that glass-eyed horses are spookier or wilder than other horses. This is simply not true. The white around the eye, or "staring" effect, often makes them *look* wilder, but the glass eye is not related to disposition. There have been many well-known horses with glass eyes.

Horses that have no pigment around the eye—those with white hair and pink eyelids—are very sensitive to sunlight irritation and cancer of the eyelids. One often sees albinos and paints like this. But the condition has nothing to do with the glass eye. If a glass-eyed horse has pigmented skin around the eye, and a tapetum lucidum in the eye, his eyes are just as good as the eye of any other horse.

There are several general principles about eye care worth mentioning:

1/ In any of these eye problems, it helps to keep the horse in a dark stall. Darkness will relieve pain and hasten healing because it rests the eye.

2/ Vitamin A is important for eye health. If this vitamin is lacking, the horse will have poor night vision and eye injuries will heal slowly. Whenever I treat an eye, I like to prescribe a feed supplement containing vitamin A. If the horse has been on a vitamin A-deficient ration (dry, bleached hay or pasture), I also give vitamin A by injection.

3/ The eye of any animal deserves the same care, the same medications, the same medical techniques that your own eyes would receive. This is no place for crude pinkeye powders, or the handful of salt treatment (care to try the latter in your own eye sometime?). A horse's damaged eye, in my opinion, should be treated with fine ophthalmic preparations and the most skilled surgical procedures. Treated in this way, the eye heals more quickly, and in many cases is saved from blindness.

4/ Don't use drugs in an eye unless you have been instructed to do so by a qualified person. The very medicine that saves one eye may destroy another. If in doubt, put the horse in a dark stall and wash the eye with a little collyrium (simple eyewash, available at most drugstores without prescription). Don't medicate an eye unless you know what you're doing. Eye medicines often have powerful and varied effects, and you don't want to risk worsening an eye problem by using some drops or ointment that you found in the medicine cabinet.

5/ A horse with a painful eye will sometimes rub it, thereby causing more damage. Cross-tie such a horse, and tranquilize him if necessary.

6/ Try to prevent eye troubles by controlling flies, giving prompt attention to any eye injury or infection, protecting the unpigmented eye from sunlight, and checking corrals and pastures for eye hazards like low-hanging tree branches.

Chronic Nasal Discharge

Horses are often seen with a persistent discharge from one or both nostrils. The patient may feel and act well otherwise. Sometimes the discharge is accompanied by a cough, snorting, or sneezing. I am talking about a situation that lasts for month after month, not for a few days or weeks as in common respiratory infections.

Chronic nasal discharge may signal benign tumors of the nasal passage, allergy, cancer, chronic infection, or a foreign body. The most common cause of such a discharge in horses, however, is infection of either the sinuses or of the guttural pouch.

The sinuses are hollow chambers within the bones of the skull. They may become infected as a result of a cold, flu, distemper, or other respiratory infection; or from an injury such as a blow to the head, or from an abscessed tooth. In most cases the discharge will come only from one nostril, because only the sinuses on that side are infected. In advanced cases, the forehead or facial bones may bulge, the eye on the involved side may squint, and the breath may have the odor of decay. Mild cases may respond well to antibiotics, although long treatment is usually required. Advanced cases may require surgical drainage. Of course, if a diseased tooth is involved, dentistry will be necessary.

Horses have an air sac on each side of the throat that communicates with the respiratory system. These sacs are called the guttural pouches. Sometimes the pouches become infected and fill with pus. Either one or both pouches may be involved. The causes of such infections are most often neglected respiratory infections, such as strangles.

Guttural pouch infection will cause a nasal discharge, especially when the head is lowered, as when grazing. The lymph nodes of the throat are also sometimes swollen. In severe cases, the swelling of the pouches may interfere with swallowing, or cause noisy breathing during exercise. The head may be cocked to one side. Infected guttural pouches may bleed. Although it is unusual, a fatal hemorrhage can occur.

There is another disease of the guttural pouch, most common in baby foals. This is called tympanitis of the pouch, and it is caused by the pouch being distended with air.

Both infection and tympanitis of the guttural pouch require surgery. This involves a delicate operation under the ear. This operation requires great skill because of the important arteries, nerves, ducts, and veins in that area. Most cases, fortunately, respond well to surgery. Early cases of guttural pouch infection may respond to antibiotics and flushing of the infected pouch. The veterinarian does this through a nasal catheter.

Strangles

Strangles is sometimes known as *distemper* or *colt distemper*. Strangles in the horse is caused by bacteria—*Streptococcus equi.* It must not be confused with dog or cat distemper, which are virus diseases and are not communicable to horses.

Strangles is found everywhere that horses live, and it can occur at any time of the year. Young horses are more susceptible, but it can hit horses at any stage of life. In recent years it has become more common in older horses, including some past 20 years of age. Moreover, a horse can contract strangles more than once. The disease is quickly spread by the nasal discharge, which is usually thick and abundant, and which remains infectious on the premises for many months.

The earliest symptoms are loss of appetite, fever, and sore throat. Later, the lymph glands of the throat swell. This often causes interference with breathing—leading to the name of the disease. In extreme cases, a tracheostomy (a surgical opening in the windpipe) may have to be performed so the patient can breathe. Eventually the swollen glands abscess. Once the abscesses drain, discharging large amounts of pus, most cases quickly recover. This usually takes a couple of weeks. However, as we shall see, some cases develop serious complications, and once in a while (about 1 or 2 percent of the time) a horse will die of strangles.

Within the veterinary profession, there are two controversies concerning strangles. One involves treatment of the disease, and the other prevention.

The streptococcus that causes strangles is very sensitive to penicillin, as well as other antibiotics and sulfa drugs. But inadequate penicillin therapy can interfere with the horse's immune response to the disease and cause a more prolonged course, or the development of chronic abscesses. For this reason, some veterinarians, and even some veterinary schools, advocate that strangles not be treated, that it be allowed to run its course until the horse spontaneously recovers. This attitude is also found on some breeding farms and stables, where it is believed that the horses simply have to "get the disease and get it over with."

I emphatically and totally disagree with this idea.

Strangles is caused by a penicillin-sensitive organism. The secret to treating strangles is to use *massive* doses of penicillin, to start using penicillin as early as possible in the course of the disease, and to continue treatment for a long-enough period. Problems arise from using doses that are too small, too infrequent, and for too short a period.

Penicillin is an inexpensive drug, and the safest of all antibiotics (unless the patient is allergic to it). I often use doses as high as 15 million units of Procaine Penicillin G daily, in a full-grown horse, and I will continue treatment for two or three or even four weeks. I've done this for more than 30 years with consistently successful results.

Why, if strangles rarely kills a horse, do I believe in such intensive and prolonged treatment? Because of the hundreds of horses I have seen with serious complications from strangles. And I have found that the complications can usually be prevented by adequate penicillin therapy.

What complications does strangles cause?

Heart disease. Strangles *frequently* causes *myocarditis.* Permanently leaky heart valves, causing a heart murmur, are common in horses, and I am certain that a common cause of this problem is *Vegetative valvular endocarditis,* a complication of untreated strangles.

Hypopyon. I have seen several colts develop this complication of strangles, wherein the eyeball fills with pus and abscesses.

Purpura hemorrhagica. This serious complication of strangles usually occurs after the horse has apparently recovered from the disease. It is a complex and serious syndrome, characterized by swellings and internal bleeding. Most cases survive, with intensive treatment, but some die regardless of what is done. Purpura used to be common in my practice years ago, when many strangles cases went untreated by the horse owners. Today it is rare in our practice because all our strangles cases receive treatment now.

Polyarthritis. A disastrous complication of strangles occurs when the bacteria invade the leg joints, causing abscessation and destruction of the joint.

Internal abscesses. Untreated strangles cases may develop abscesses in the chest or in the abdomen. If diagnosed early, such cases can survive, with intensive antibiotic treatment. However, if such an abscess ruptures internally, it will cause the death of the horse. This may happen many weeks after the patient has apparently recovered from what may have appeared to be a mild case of strangles.

Bastard strangles. This condition is a chronic problem, occurring after the acute stages of strangles have subsided, characterized by the formation of many small scattered abscesses in various parts of the body. In my experience, bastard strangles does *not* occur if acute strangles cases are treated adequately, and that means *prompt, massive* doses of penicillin for a *long* time.

Guttural pouch infection. Horses have a unique structure deep in the throat, just below the ear. On each side there is a "pocket" that communicates with the eustachian tube. These are called guttural pouches. During strangles, these pouches sometimes fill with pus, causing a chronic and troublesome problem called empyema of the guttural pouch. Similarly, some horses with strangles develop chronic infections of the sinus cavities, within the skull.

Brain abscesses. It is rare, but once in a while a strangles abscess will develop in a horse's brain, a catastrophic complication.

The second controversy about strangles concerns the use of the vaccine *Strangles Bacterin* to prevent the disease. Many veterinarians, and some veterinary schools, are reluctant to recommend strangles immunization to horse owners because: 1/ The vaccine is not a highly effective vaccine, protecting perhaps 75 percent of the inoculated horses for 6 to 12 months; 2/ The vaccine itself can cause problems. These range from severe swelling to an occasional abscess at the injection site, to a rare purpura-type reaction.

Until recently, I would agree with the above, and I did *not* routinely recommend strangles immunization. However, there are improved new vaccines available that have largely eliminated the problems mentioned. The new vaccines contain a substance called M-protein, isolated from the streptococcus that causes strangles, and free from the portions of the bacteria that cause the reactions in the older vaccine.

In my practice, we have used thousands of doses of the new vaccine with no more problems than we experience from other vaccines (tetanus, influenza, rhinopneumonitis, etc.). Most important, we see a great reduction in the incidence of strangles, especially on breeding farms where the disease is an annual problem.

I feel that great progress has been made against strangles since I entered the veterinary profession in 1956. We can effectively prevent the disease, especially on an epidemic basis, by regularly immunizing horses with the newer vaccines. We can effectively treat the disease. In fact—if strangles is attacked vigorously during its very early stages, as in the first 24 hours—the disease can be aborted with penicillin. More important, with proper treatment, we can prevent some of the nasty crippling and even fatal complications of strangles.

Equine Encephalitis

Summertime means mosquitoes in many parts of the country. Mosquitoes carry the virus of equine sleeping sickness or equine encephalitis. Don't confuse this disease with African sleeping sickness, an entirely different malady carried by the tsetse fly.

Horses are not the only victims of viral encephalitis. Many other animals and birds can contract it. Encephalitis may be carried by pheasants and pigeons. Most important, humans can catch encephalitis. There are periodic outbreaks in humans in various parts of the United States. However, humans and horses cannot transmit the disease directly to one another. Apparently, humans and horses are both dead-end hosts. The mosquito host is responsible for the spread of the disease, to the best of our knowledge. It is possible that other insects may also be involved. Incidentally, the disease used to be called equine encephalomyelitis, but encephalitis or sleeping sickness is easier to say and spell.

There are several kinds of equine sleeping sickness. In the United States, we presently have eastern equine encephalitis and western equine encephalitis. In 1971 we had an outbreak of Venezuelan equine encephalitis.

The virus damages the brain and spinal cord, and the symptoms seen are due to the damage to these organs. Depending on the part of the brain destroyed, we might see paralysis of the jaws, grinding of the teeth, twitching of muscles, insane movements, excitement, or paralysis. Frequently there is the drowsy stupidity that gives the disease its common name.

Not all horses die of sleeping sickness, but many of those that recover suffer permanent mental damage. Like other viruses that attack the central nervous system (human polio, dog distemper, rabies, etc.), sleeping sickness is easier to prevent than to treat. In fact, there is no specific treatment for such diseases. These viruses are not affected by antibiotics.

As is the case with most diseases caused by viruses, no specific cure has yet been discovered. Fortunately, however, there are excellent equine vaccines available against both eastern and western encephalitis. Two injections are given one to four weeks apart.

Because these diseases are primarily carried by mosquitoes, the best time to vaccinate is in the spring. Obviously, a mosquito control program will help reduce the incidence of sleeping sickness in areas where the disease occurs.

Another virus that attacks the brain is *rabies.* As nearly everybody knows, rabies is caused by a virus that is found in the saliva of rabid animals. The disease is transmitted by biting, and when the virus reaches the brain, death inevitably follows. Horses can and do get rabies, though only a few cases a year are reported in the United States. Horses are usually exposed by being bitten by rabid dogs or wild animals. Afflicted horses show the usual symptoms of mental derangement, viciousness, inability to swallow, paralysis, convulsions, and finally, death. In order to make a positive diagnosis of rabies, the animal's brain must be saved for a laboratory examination; so under no circumstances should a horse suspected of having rabies be killed by shooting him in the head.

A vaccine labelled specifically for horses is available and is being widely used.

Snakebite

Poisonous snakes are found scattered throughout North America, and they are especially common in some areas where large numbers of saddle horses are found, such as the southwestern states.

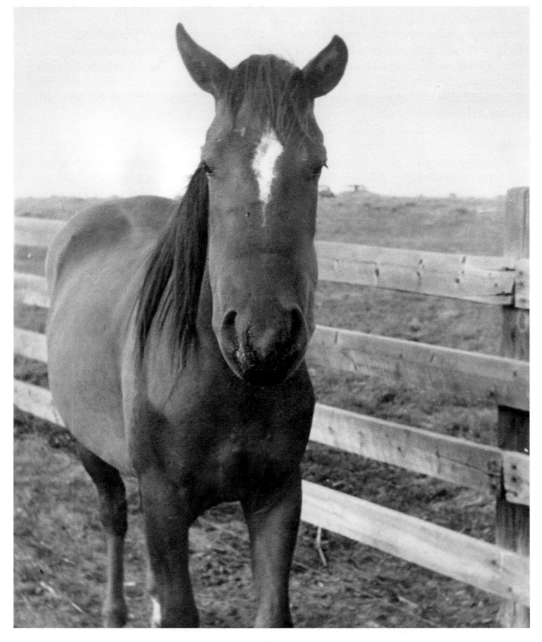

It is not unusual for a horse to be bitten by a poisonous snake, and the horseman ought to know a little bit about the proper treatment of snakebite.

Occasionally the rider will actually see the horse being bitten. If the bite is on an extremity, apply a tourniquet above the wound; that is, between the fang marks and the heart. Loosen the tourniquet every 15 minutes. Move it upward as the swelling progresses. Incision and suction may be used promptly after the bite. Avoid moving the horse and excite him as little as possible. Call a veterinarian as soon as you can.

More often the horse will be found in the pasture with a swollen leg or nose. Bites around the head are especially dangerous to horses because severe swelling of the nose or throat may interfere with breathing, shut off the animal's air supply, and he will then die of asphyxia, or lack of oxygen. In such cases a tracheostomy may be necessary. This is an emergency operation in which the windpipe is exposed through a throat incision, and a tube put in through which the animal breathes.

Most cases of snakebite in horses are not fatal. Even without treatment most horses will survive, although this varies from one region of the country to another. However, the administration of various drugs, such as cortisone, antivenin, and penicillin will greatly reduce the animal's suffering. Proper treatment will prevent complications, return the horse to use much more quickly, greatly reduce tissue sloughing afterwards, and may prevent death. The veterinarian will also inject the horse with tetanus antitoxin, or tetanus toxoid, whichever is appropriate. Tetanus immunization is a vital part of snakebite treatment. Sometimes surgical drainage of severely swollen areas is necessary.

Beware the advice of well-meaning but unqualified laymen who will recommend all sorts of primitive, useless, if not harmful, remedies. The treatment of snakebite in a horse is essentially the same as in humans. To do less for the horse is both inhumane and impractical.

Cancer

Like all animals, horses can die of cancer. If cancer is detected early and treated properly, many of these deaths can be avoided. Most of the rules in human cancer detection also apply to animals, including horses.

Cancer is a sneaky, insidious disease. In the early stages it is usually painless, and therefore it often does not alarm the person involved until it may be too late.

A cancer is a malignant tumor. It is a growing mass of tissue that can destroy its host in two ways. First it infiltrates. That is, it grows and grows, spreading roots out in any direction until its size mechanically interferes with the organs it is growing on. Secondly, a cancer may metastasize. This means that it can send out seed cells that take root elsewhere in the body and start to grow. Thus, an intestinal cancer may spread to the liver, or a skin cancer of the face may spread to the lymph nodes of the throat.

Not all cancers metastasize. Some only infiltrate. And, of those that do metastasize, some do early, and others late. Cancers vary in rate of growth. Some kill in weeks, others take years. Some cancers are easily curable. For others, no treatment is effective.

The veterinarian cannot make a positive diagnosis of cancer by simply examining the animal. He may *suspect* the disease, but a positive diagnosis can only be made by *biopsy*—that is, by microscopic examination of a bit of the tumor tissue.

As you all know, we still have a great deal to learn regarding the cause and cure of cancers.

Any kind of cancer may be found in any animal. But every species of animal has certain cancers to which it is prone. In fact, the susceptibility to cancer often varies with the breed or color of the animal. These observations apply to the horse.

SQUAMOUS CELL CARCINOMA

Horses with unpigmented eyelids are very susceptible to a type of skin cancer known as *squamous cell carcinoma*. It may occur in any white-faced or pale-skinned horse. Albinos, Paints, Appaloosas, and palominos are commonly affected.

This kind of cancer is caused by the irritating effect of sunlight on skin or membranes unprotected by hair or pigment. In my practice in sunny California, I see many cases of squamous cell carcinoma of the eyelid.

The color of the horse does not increase susceptibility if the eyelids are pigmented. In other words, a white horse is not necessarily vulnerable if he has black eyelids. The skin pigment, melanin, protects against sunlight. For example, we often see a paint horse with one eye surrounded with dark skin and the other eye surrounded by unpigmented pink skin. It is the unpigmented side that will have the cancer.

Sometimes we see an eye in which all but a small area of lid is pigmented, perhaps not much more than a quarter of an inch long, and a carcinoma develops on that small unprotected area.

Horses are not the only animals that develop squamous cell carcinoma of the skin from sunlight irritation. It even occurs in humans. Cats with white ears often get this type of cancer at the tips of the ears where there is little hair to shield against the sun. Collie dogs and related breeds sometimes have an inherited allergy to sunlight that causes a skin condition called "Collie nose" at the unpigmented junction of the nose with the hairy bridge of the nose. After a few years, this condition may turn into a squamous cell carcinoma. Horses can develop the same cancer at other hairless areas if unpigmented, such as under the tail or around the mouth or genitalia.

In animals, squamous cell carcinoma is seen most often in the eyes of white-faced Hereford cattle. "Cancer eye" is a familiar problem to cattlemen, especially in arid sunny regions, or at high altitudes where the sun's rays are undiluted and often reflected off the snow.

In horses this kind of cancer rarely appears without warning. Usually the eyelid has a long history of irritation, sunburn, and excessive tear flow. Often a pre-cancerous ulcerated sore appears on the lid. The inner corner of the lower lid is most often involved, but any portion of the upper or lower lid may be, or even the nictitating membrane (the "third eyelid" at the inner corner of an animal's eye).

Once the lesion becomes cancerous, it will not heal without treatment. It will continue to grow and spread, sometimes rapidly and sometimes very slowly, until it eventually kills the horse.

Fortunately, if caught early enough, most squamous cell carcinoma of the horse's eyelids can be cured. Four kinds of treatment are effective. They are:

1/ Operation (cutting the cancer out surgically).

2/ Irradiation (treating the cancer with X-ray, radium, strontium 90, or other radioactive materials).

3/ Injection into the cancer of an anti-cancer drug called by various trade names, including Ribigen and Nomagen.

4/ Cauterization (treatment with heat, particularly with high-frequency electrical fulguration).

In the author's experience, the last method has been enormously successful. Frequently two of the three methods are combined, especially on larger lesions.

On some larger lesions, a considerable portion of eyelid must be removed, necessitating plastic surgery to restore the lid. Where the cancer is on the third eyelid, that structure can be simply amputated without noticeably disfiguring the horse.

If you own a horse with an unpigmented eye, you should take certain precautions to prevent eyelid cancer. All of these precautions are designed to reduce the amount of sunlight hitting the eye.

1/ Keep the horse out of the sun as much as possible by stabling during daylight hours, providing shady corrals, and taking extra precautions during the long summer days. Remember that sunlight can be reflected off light-colored surfaces.

2/ Have the horse wear a fly net over his eyes when he's not being ridden.

3/ Protect the unpigmented eyelid with mascara, or a dark blue pinkeye spray that is made for cattle (but paint it on a horse, don't spray it). Or darken the area with a black felt marking pencil or black makeup. You may even have the lid tattooed, but this may have to be redone periodically.

4/ If the horse already has a sore on the lid, have it examined by a veterinarian promptly. Don't wait until it is too late.

The same cancer is often found on other unpigmented and thinly haired areas, such as the sheath. In fact the sheath and penis of the horse are common locations for several types of cancer. Keeping the sheath clean may help

Keeping the sheath clean may help to prevent some of these cancers because we believe they are the result of prolonged irritation due to accumulated debris.

73

to prevent some of these cancers because we believe they are the result of prolonged irritation due to accumulated debris.

MELANOMA

This common growth is a black-pigmented type of malignancy. It may occur in any horse, but is usually found in old gray horses. Most melanomas are located in the perineal region, under or close to the root of the tail.

LEUKEMIA

This is a cancer of the blood cells. There is no cure, but a dramatic temporary improvement often follows treatment with cortisone or chemotherapy.

SARCOID

Horses are sometimes afflicted with a unique tumor called *equine sarcoid*. It has been diagnosed in horses of every size, breed, age, and color and has been found in many parts of the world. It is a skin tumor and is most common on the head, neck, shoulders, chest, and legs, but is sometimes found on the skin over the ribs or reproductive organs. The ear is a common site.

Sarcoids, in general, take one of two forms. They may appear as flat, gray, wart-like lesions, usually one-half to two inches in diameter; or they may take the form of "proud flesh," especially those that appear on the legs. The latter type of equine sarcoid can reach enormous sizes and can be very discouraging to treat. Leg wounds often develop sarcoids.

Many authorities believe that the tumor is caused by the virus that causes warts on cattle. Others have reason to believe that another virus is responsible. For many years, however, nearly all veterinarians have felt sure that a virus was definitely involved. Experimental work in Colorado (where equine sarcoid is common) supports the virus theory.

There are several points I'd like to emphasize about equine sarcoids. First, do not confuse the ordinary seed warts or blood warts with sarcoid. These warts, so often found on the lips or nose of a young horse, are caused by a virus, but will disappear eventually—even if they are not treated. Second, realize that it takes a pathologist's biopsy to *positively* diagnose a sarcoid. There are many other lesions a horse can get that look similar to sarcoid.

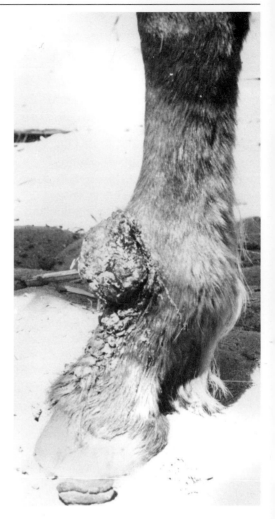

Third, take care of wounds, particularly wire cuts on the legs. I believe that prompt and *correct* treatment, and the use of sterile pressure dressings on leg wounds greatly inhibit the development of the big, granulating sarcoids.

When I was a student, back in the fifties, there was no effective treatment for sarcoids. If they were surgically removed, they often grew back in a more horrible form than before. Then, in 1968, at the American Association of Equine Practitioners meeting in Philadelphia, two successful forms of treatment were announced. One was cryosurgery, a freezing technique. The other was the use of fluorouracil solution, an anti-cancer chemical applied with wet packs. Then another chemical, polophyllin, was reported to be effective against sarcoids. I started using Efudex cream, a fluorouracil compound for human skin cancer, with consistently good results. This prescription drug is applied to the tumor, once daily, without bandaging or rubbing it in, for a month. The person applying the Efudex cream must wear protective gloves because it is an irritant, and for a while, the tumor will look worse. Two months later I re-examine the tumor and if it isn't completely gone, I treat it a second time. I have also removed large sarcoids surgically, and then used Efudex cream to prevent recurrence, and it works extremely well.

More recently, two new forms of treatment have been introduced. I have used both with success, sometimes combining both treatments. One is the use of the thermoprobe, an instrument that kills the tumor cells with heat. The other is by means of injecting an anti-cancer drug containing trexalose dimycolate and a mycobacterial cell-wall fraction. This drug is an immuno-stimulant and is quite effective against certain types of cancer and is equally effective in removing equine sarcoids.

So, in the last two decades, several very effective methods of treating equine sarcoids have been developed.

Urinary Problems

Horsemen of the old school are often preoccupied with the horse's kidney function. "It's his kidneys, Doc," is a common lament. The shelves of tack shops sometimes contain kidney stimulants, and some of them are a bit dangerous.

Why do horsemen worry about the horse's kidneys? There are several possible explanations. Horses with colic or any abdominal pain will often stretch as if to urinate, whereas in reality they are stretching to relieve pain.

Any animal, when sick or injured, will show a slowdown in urine production. This can be from dehydration, or the body's effort to conserve fluids by retaining urine. That's why the physician says, "Stay in bed and drink plenty of liquids."

Horses often suffer back pain. Since the kidneys are in the loin area, they are often unjustly blamed for the pain.

Several diseases of the horse cause abnormally colored urine. This occurs in azoturia and in jaundice. The horseman, noting the obvious change, blames the kidneys, whereas the real cause is elsewhere in the body. Of course, in such diseases, the kidney might be damaged, but it is secondary. The primary problem is still elsewhere.

Actually, urinary disease is rare in the horse. But it is common in humans, dogs, cats, and in ruminant animals like cattle and sheep.

Once in a while we see a horse with bladder or kidney stones, or a horse with an infection of the urinary tract. Tumors of the urinary system in horses are very unusual. Sudan grass has been known to cause cystitis (bladder inflammation) in horses.

Although the urinary organs of the horse are seldom diseased, the urine itself is frequently abnormal. The color of the urine can be abnormal secondarily to some diseases. For example, a jaundiced horse will have orange urine, and a horse with phenothiazine poisoning or with certain blood diseases will have red urine. Azoturia, a common muscle disease in horses, will often cause myoglobinuria. This refers to the presence of myoglobin, a muscle pigment in the urine. It will cause brown urine that looks much like coffee.

Many inexperienced people are frightened by the appearance of perfectly normal horse urine. Unlike the urine of most animals, horse urine contains a lot of mucus that is secreted by special cells in the kidney. The mucus content, which varies in quantity, causes horse urine to have a high viscosity. In other words, it has a kind of slimy or oily quality.

Horse urine is also normally turbid, or cloudy in appearance. This is especially true of the last part of the urine when the bladder is emptied. In most animals, turbidity or cloudiness is a sign of trouble, but it is quite normal in the horse. The turbidity is due to the presence of minerals in the urine, especially calcium carbonate. Often these minerals precipitate as white salts on the ground, again causing needless alarm in the owner.

Horse urine contains a lot of nitrogen waste compounds, such as ammonia. In a poorly ventilated stable, the ammonia fumes can make one's eyes water, and the poor horse has to live in that atmosphere all the time.

So, horse urine looks different, smells different, and even feels different, but that doesn't mean the horse is sick. Urinary disease is rare in the horse, but it can occur and does occur. If a real abnormality is seen, discuss it with your veterinarian. An examination and a urinalysis will determine if a problem is really present.

Kidney Trouble

One of the most common diseases attributed to the horse, especially around stables and the racetrack, is kidney trouble. Many horsemen blame the kidneys for almost every ailment that befalls a horse. Some horse owners still routinely administer kidney stimulants to their horses. When a horse suffers colic, lumbar back pain, myositis, anemia, parasitism, or any unexplained illness, we so often hear the remark, "It's his kidneys, Doc."

In truth, the horse is exceptionally immune to kidney disorders when compared to other domestic animals. Veterinarians in equine practice may see thousands of sick horses annually, and only find one or two cases of kidney disease.

The kidney is an organ essential to life. Horses are born with two kidneys, located in their abdomen under the lumbar spine. Large blood vessels supply the kidney, which selectively removes certain substances from the blood and, from these substances, it forms urine. The urine passes from the kidney to the bladder through a tube called a ureter. The bladder periodically empties when the horse urinates.

The kidney has many important functions. It maintains the normalcy of blood plasma by removing waste products, removing certain salts, eliminating water, and disposing of many foreign substances—including most drugs. Nature has been generous in that the body has more kidney than it really needs. Thus much of the kidney can be destroyed by disease and yet life can go on with the remaining kidney tissue carrying the load. Even the loss of an entire kidney is not fatal, if the other is healthy and functioning.

Disorders elsewhere in the body may affect the nature of the urine. For example, an illness may result in less urine formation simply because the kidney is trying to conserve water to prevent dehydration of the entire body. So don't be alarmed because a sick horse doesn't "pass water." It doesn't mean that his kidneys are necessarily diseased. Certain drugs and body pigments may give the urine an abnormal color. This doesn't mean that the horse's kidneys are in trouble. In fact, it indicates that they are doing the job they are supposed to do.

If you are concerned about the health of your horse's kidneys, two simple tests will quickly reveal any malfunction. These are a urinalysis, and a blood test. Unless these tests, or a veterinarian's examination, reveal positive kidney disease, don't ever give your horse a kidney stimulant. Most of the nostrums sold for this purpose are antiquated compounds of vegetable juices or chemicals. Some of them can actually damage the kidney. When kidney stimulants *are* needed, we have many new, safe drugs available to us.

The kidney of the horse *can* be afflicted with stones, tumors, infections, poisons, and degenerative diseases. All of these conditions are serious, and the horse with such a disease is a very sick animal.

So don't jump to the conclusion that a sore back or attack of colic means kidney trouble. Remember that the best kidney stimulant is an abundant supply of fresh water and free-choice white salt. These, along with regular exercise and a wholesome diet, are pretty good insurance against your horse ever suffering from a kidney ailment.

Ear Problems

Compared to some other animals, horses rarely have trouble with their ears—probably because in domesticating the horse we have tampered very little with the natural anatomy of the ear. By contrast, look at the dog. All wild dogs (fox, wolf, coyote, jackal, dingo, etc.) have an erect, open ear. But many domestic dogs have pendulous ears, or ears that are small, or constricted, or filled with thick hair. Consequently, dogs suffer from many ear diseases, compared to horses.

Nevertheless, horses *do* have a few ear problems. One of the most common is infestation by ear ticks. These parasites invade the ear canal of horses (and other animals) and cause great discomfort. The horse will shake his head, hold it to one side, and lay the ear back on the affected side. He may resent the ear being handled. Ear ticks are easily killed by instilling appropriate medication into the ear. Such medicines can be prescribed by your veterinarian.

The normal ear secretes wax. When an ear is irritated, as by an infection or by ticks, excessive wax may form. It is difficult to remove this discharge with swabs or instruments. The horse will usually not cooperate. There are, however, solvents that can easily be put into the ear that dissolve ear wax, allowing the horse to shake it out. Such preparations are called cerumenolytic agents, and are familiar to most veterinarians. Tick-killing chemicals may be mixed with these solvents.

Many horses develop vices about their ears. Some are ear-shy and will not allow one or both ears to be handled, as when bridling for example. This vice is due to training errors or omissions. *Earing* a horse to restrain him, or applying a twitch to the ear will not cause ear-shyness, *if the restraint is properly applied.* Attacking the horse suddenly and trying to pull an ear off will make any horse ear-shy.

When earing a horse, work slowly, gently, and gradually. Do not pull or twist the ear. Merely apply intermittent and powerful pressure with the tips of the fingers. When completed, release the ear gradually, and finish by gently massaging the ear. The last memory the horse has should be a pleasant one. Then he will not fear your hand near his ear. The ears should be frequently handled and rubbed so the horse is used to it. Earing a horse as described takes a strong grip and short fingernails.

Another ear vice is what we used to call "sour-ear" back on the ranch. The horse acts as if he has a tick in the ear, but *only* when being ridden. I've seen horses develop this vice as a result of a flapping headstall strap, or a jingling buckle, or because of a cranky disposition. If the horse really has ticks, he will not show the symptoms only when under saddle.

Horses often get flat, gray, wart-like lesions in the ears called aural plaques. These are persistent, and usually bother the owner more than they do the horse. We do not recommend treatment unless the problem is severe. However, some-

times these plaques get fly-bitten. The daily application of a fly repellent cream or ointment will help.

Other tumors can affect the ear, including some malignancies. I have seen sarcoid in the ear; and in gray horses, melanoma on or near the ear is rather common.

In cold climates, frostbitten ears are not unusual. Many, many horses have had their ears frozen off, especially when pastured in the open—a common practice in the western range country.

Of course, the ears are subjected to wounds many times. We've all seen split-eared horses. This disfigurement can be avoided if the wound is surgically repaired.

We should also mention the "ear-tooth," or dentigerous cyst. This is one of nature's mistakes—a congenital deformity wherein a misplaced tooth develops somewhere near the ear, usually at its base. A draining hole or fistula forms from the tooth, discharging to the surface. The only cure is surgery.

Infection of the external ear *(otitis externa* or "canker") and infection of the middle ear *(otitis media),* both of which are so common in dogs, are much less common in horses. However, they do occur and require veterinary attention. Otitis externa manifests discharge and a foul odor. Otitis media will cause head tilting, dizziness, and sometimes a loss of balance.

There are several conditions to which the horse is prone that do not involve the ear itself, but which are so intimately involved with the ear that they deserve to be mentioned here.

Parotitis is swelling and inflammation of the parotid salivary gland, just below the ear.

Disease of the guttural pouch can also cause swelling beneath the ear. This structure, peculiar to horses, is a blind pouch or sac that opens into the eustachian tube of the inner ear. It may get infected and fill with pus; or in foals, it sometimes distends with air, causing a condition called tympanitis of the guttural pouch.

Both parotitis and guttural pouch disease are problems requiring the attention of a veterinarian.

This is one of nature's mistakes— a congenital deformity wherein a misplaced tooth develops somewhere near the ear, usually at its base.

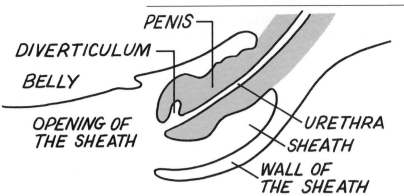

PENIS

DIVERTICULUM

BELLY

OPENING OF
THE SHEATH

URETHRA

SHEATH

WALL OF
THE SHEATH

Cleaning the Sheath

An often-neglected, but important part of good horse management is the periodic cleaning of the gelding's sheath. Debris accumulates within this organ, and if not removed, it will eventually cause irritation.

This irritation, in time, can lead to many complications. These include infection and ulceration of the sheath or penis, swelling, interference with the passage of urine, and occasionally, the eventual development of cancer. Cancer of the sheath and penis is a common malignancy in the horse, and lack of cleanliness is probably the reason for this.

The debris that accumulates within the sheath comes from several sources. Mud, dust, and bedding account for some of it. The precipitation of minerals within the urine also contributes. But most of the putty-like debris is secreted by the horse himself. This secretion is called *smegma*.

Some geldings require cleaning of the sheath as often as once a month. Most horses need to be cleaned less often. Certainly *every* gelding should be cleaned *at least* once a year. Some horsemen do this job themselves, and others have their veterinarians do it. This is a good chore to have done when the veterinarian is out for some other routine work such as vaccinating, worming, or dentistry. Don't wait until after infection develops, or the sheath is swollen, or the horse is unable to urinate.

To clean the sheath in the simplest way possible, I do not attempt to get the horse to "drop," or extend the penis. Instead, I ease a garden hose into the sheath and allow it to run with moderate pressure, using no nozzle and a smooth-ended hose. Simply irrigating the sheath in this manner will wash away a lot of debris, and this can be done frequently; say at weekly intervals. This procedure causes no discomfort to the horse (unless the water is awfully cold) and if he is well-mannered he should not object.

Many horses, however, will object and a bit of training may be necessary. Start by getting your horse used to a hose. If he fears it, use a slow trickle on a hot day. Start with his feet, and very, very gradually work up to the rest of his body. Once he learns to enjoy being hosed off, start directing the stream of water at his sheath, using low pressure. Eventually he will allow you to insert the hose into the sheath and he will tolerate a moderately forceful stream of water.

At least once a year, a more thorough cleaning will be necessary. In fact, some horses require thorough cleaning two or three or four times a year. Once in a while we find a gelding that has a lot of secretion and has to be cleaned every few weeks. The secretions combine with sweat, dust, and dirt to form tenacious debris within the sheath.

It is not necessary to exteriorize the penis unless specific lesions need to be treated.

First, irrigate the sheath. If the opening of the sheath is held tightly closed around the hose the sheath will quickly balloon up with water. When the opening to the sheath is released, all of the water gushes out, carrying out a lot of debris. The inside of the sheath is now completely wet. Next take a handful of soap, and carry it into the sheath.

You can carry in a palmful of liquid soap (I always use Joy), or a bar of soap, or a small soapy sponge. Now lather everything within the sheath very thoroughly. If the horse is very dirty, you can bring out handfuls of debris. Soap up your hand first. The lather will serve as lubrication, and make it easier to work the hand all the way to the back of the sheath. Using lots of soap, wash the entire inside of the sheath.

Many horsemen neglect the following procedure when cleaning a horse's sheath: Just within the urethra, which is the tube through which the urine leaves the body, lies a blind pouch or diverticulum. Smegma accumulates within this pouch, often forming a stone or "bean."

Removing this is a very important part of the sheath-cleaning procedure, because it is this stone that causes urinary obstruction. Usually the stone is soft enough to be broken up and removed with the finger.

When cleaning the sheath it is important that all parts and folds within it be included.

One word of caution: The debris being removed teems with bacteria. If one has breaks in the skin, contact with this material can cause a severe infection.

Cleaning the sheath is not a pleasant job, even for the veterinarian. It is hard to do wearing gloves, and the odor of the debris is very difficult to remove from one's hands. But the importance of doing the job cannot be over-emphasized.

After cleaning the sheath it is very important to rinse repeatedly and remove all traces of soap. If soap is left in the sheath it may cause irritation.

Back Problems

Do you know which three creatures in the world have the most back trouble? The answer: humans, Dachshunds, and horses. We humans are prone to back trouble because we walk on our hind legs. We've only been doing this for a short while (from an evolutionary standpoint), and the strain on our back often causes it to break down.

Dachshunds are a breed of dog selectively bred for their short legs and long back. In dogs with such backs, back trouble is extremely common. Apparently the back is architecturally unstable, and that, combined with degenerative changes, leads to trouble.

Horses walk on all fours, and they have a well-constructed back. But nature never intended the horse to carry weight on his back, at high speed, over jumps, and during sudden starts, stops, and turns. No wonder horses are prone to back trouble.

When a human gets back trouble, the diagnosis is relatively simple. The patient complains of pain—in his back. Finding the *cause* of the back pain is another story, one which we won't attempt to discuss.

When the dog gets back trouble, the problem is only slightly more difficult.

The dog will cry when his back is pressed, has trouble going up stairs, and so on. The veterinarian performs some tests to make sure that the trouble is really in the back, and most of the time lesions will be visible on X-rays.

The horse, now, is a problem. Not that a horse won't show signs of back pain, because he will. He may be reluctant to work, may refuse to jump, refuse to turn left or right, cheat when roping, etc. He may act "cold-backed" when being saddled, act "cinch-bound," rear, lie down, hump up, or travel stiff behind. The problem is, the horseman usually accounts for such behavior with the wrong explanation. He may decide that the horse's behavior is due to a vice (which is possible, of course). He may decide that the horse is "tied-up," or needs a laxative. Often he thinks that the horse has kidney trouble, and wants to give him a kidney stimulant. Actually, horses are more resistant to kidney trouble than any other animal. Meanwhile, the poor horse is simply suffering from back trouble.

When we say back trouble, we can be talking about many different problems. The back consists of the vertebrae, which are a chain of spinal bones. Through this chain runs the spinal cord, and from the cord come many vital nerves. The bones articulate with each other by means of a series of joints, and are separated by the intervertebral discs. These are shock-absorbing cushions between each vertebra. All of this is held together by a system of ligaments, and the back can bend up, down, or to either side when pulled by a complicated arrangement of muscles that extend along its length.

Any of these structures can be damaged. Discs can rupture, bones can break or dislocate, ligaments can stretch or tear, and so can the muscles. The muscles can also go into painful spasms from strain. If the spinal cord or nerves are pinched, then the horse has pain, and he can also have partial or complete paralysis of the part supplied by that nerve. From chronic injury, the articulations can become damaged. Then the horse has arthritis of the back.

A machine of enormous power is necessary to X-ray a horse's back. Diagnostic back pictures are not possible with the portable X-ray machines used by most equine practitioners. So you can see that an exact diagnosis is often impossible. In fact, it is an accomplishment simply to recognize that the problem does, indeed, lie in the back. Then appropriate treatment can be given. Most cases of simple *sore back* in horses are due to strain, and respond very well to medication. There are rare cases that involve the bone, and some of these can be helped with surgery. Naturally, rest is always helpful.

We have spent most of our discussion on conditions that affect the lumbar area primarily. This area, corresponding to the lower back in man, lies from about the cantle area of the saddle back to the rump. Most of the sprains, strains, and common back problems in horses are found in this part of the back. But the back begins at the withers, and goes clear to the tail, so we must mention several other common back problems.

Fistula of the withers. This is an infected draining bursitis of the withers, caused by bruising, and often by an ill-fitting saddle. If not arrested early, it will lead to a nasty, deep infection requiring radical surgery. Call your veterinarian promptly.

Sit-fast. These hard, skin lesions of the back are similar to a corn on your toe. Like a corn, they are caused by pressure; in this case from the saddle. Prevent them by using clean, thick saddle blankets and a well-fitting saddle. Also, ride in balance. If you slouch in the saddle and don't ride "with the horse," it is hard on his back.

Saddle sores and cinch sores. It is not humane to ride a horse with a sore back or one suffering from sores or galls under the cinch. Moreover, if such sores are repeatedly injured and not allowed to heal, they may develop thick scar tissue which then becomes a permanent problem instead of a temporary one.

There are a multitude of remedies on the market for saddle sores. Horsemen are always looking for some kind of medication to treat a sore with, so that it will heal while they continue to ride the horse. For this purpose there are many kinds of lotions, ointments, and powders, plus a variety of home remedies. But, as a matter of fact, all that is needed to heal such a sore is time and rest. If the horse is not ridden, the sore will heal. Of course, if infection is present, a medication to clear up the infection is helpful. But basically, these sores will heal if they are simply not reinjured by riding the horse.

No horseman likes to lay up a horse. And, saddle and cinch sores are disfiguring blemishes, and certainly uncomfortable for the horse. So, obviously, the best way to handle this problem—or *any* health problem—is to prevent it. It is always better, and usually easier, to prevent a disease than it is to cure it.

To prevent sores, we have to understand what causes them. Most of us simply assume that the saddle or the cinch *rubs* a raw spot on the skin, but this is not usually the case. If saddle sores were due to rubbing (chafing), then a loosely cinched saddle would cause sores more readily than a tightly cinched saddle, and such is usually not the case.

Now chafing *can* cause sores, as for example when the ring of a cinch (especially a corroded or rusty cinch ring) chafes the movable skin behind the shoulder of the horse. But this type of sore is easily controlled with a little soft padding to reduce friction. A woolskin pad can be fitted to prevent a chafing cinch ring, and other chafed areas can be similarly protected.

A lot of us also think that heat, built up under the saddle, *scalds* the skin and causes the sores. And, as a matter of fact, heat can cause inflammation of the skin—a heat rash—and make a horse's back very sore. This kind of saddle sore is prevented by good, thick, porous saddle blankets or pads that allow some air circulation under the saddle. Even more important, remove the saddle on long rides, or simply raise the skirts to let air under the saddle and allow the skin to be cooled by the evaporation of sweat.

But neither chafing nor heat cause most saddle sores. Instead, the most common cause is *pressure*. Pressure deprives the living cells of the skin of blood. Deprived of blood, the cell dies. If enough cells die, a sore results. Medically, the death of tissue in this manner is known as pressure necrosis.

We can give you many other examples of pressure necrosis. The bed sores that develop in bed-ridden people are due to pressure necrosis. A horse with a leg bandage or a cast that's too tight may develop pressure necrosis under the dressing. A heavy bosal on a hackamore usually makes a horse's nose sore by chafing, but if left on too long, pressure necrosis may develop under the bosal.

Realizing that pressure necrosis causes most saddle sores changed our concepts of how to prevent them. Which saddle distributes pressure better: a small, round-skirted saddle or a big, square-skirted one? Too tight a cinch cuts off the blood supply to skin cells. Does the fork of your saddle fit the shape of your horse's withers, distributing your weight over as large an area as possible, or does all the pressure come on a small area on either side of the withers?

Is your cinch wide, soft, and clean? Do you ride sitting up straight, with some of your weight in the stirrups, thereby transmitting your weight to the entire saddletree? Or do you ride loose in the stirrups, slouched back against the cantle, throwing all your weight on the horse's loins? If so, don't be surprised to find pressure sores under the back of the saddle when you dismount.

Use a saddle that fits your horse's back. Pad it well with clean blankets and pads. It is my firm opinion that synthetic saddle blankets and pads contribute to many back problems. I advocate the use of animal hair padding under a saddle, such as a good woolen saddle blanket, wool or hair felt pads, and real sheepskin. Put everything on a clean back. Cinch up snugly, but don't cut the horse in two. If the horse, the terrain, or roping demands it, use wide roping cinches, a back cinch, a breast collar, or a crupper . . . anything so you don't have to over-cinch.

Sit up when you ride, with weight in your stirrups, not back against the cantle. Loosen the cinch when you dismount, and don't hesitate to unsaddle on a long ride and let a little air onto the surface of the horse's skin, and a little blood into the deeper layers of his skin.

Botulism

Botulism is the most serious form of food poisoning. It is caused by eating a toxin (a poisonous substance) that develops in spoiled food that happens to be contaminated by a bacteria known as *Clostridium botulinum.*

This germ means no harm. It is a common organism that grows in soil. When, however, it finds its way into spoiling food, it produces a metabolic waste product that happens to be extremely poisonous to higher forms of animal life. It has been said that a single drop of botulinum toxin diluted into a reservoir could destroy a half-million people. This toxin, in fact, is the most poisonous substance known.

Botulism is not rare. Many people die every year from it, usually as a result of eating improperly prepared home-canned vegetables. Contaminated meats and meat products are another common cause of human botulism, especially in countries with poor meat sanitation and inspection.

In chickens and ducks, botulism is called "limberneck." I have seen it in chickens fed rotting lettuce; and it is common in ducks and other waterfowl when decomposing vegetation along the shore supports the growth of clostridium botulinum. Cattle and sheep have been known to develop botulism from licking and chewing at dead animals. They do this if they lack phosphorus in their diets.

Hay containing dead animals has been known to cause botulism. Please understand that not all dead animals contain the botulism germ. It is just that any decomposing organic material can support its growth under the right conditions. In the mink industry, the feeding of spoiled fish has caused many botulism deaths.

In horses, botulism occurs most often as a result of spoiled hay. The drouthy winter of 1974 was the only winter I practiced in California in which I failed to see at least one case of botulism in horses. All of our rain occurs in the winter, and a lot of hay gets wet during the rainy season. The wet hay spoils and if eaten by a horse, produces occasional cases of botulism. Every case I have seen in a horse, mule, or donkey has proven fatal.

Affected horses show progressive paralysis, often starting with the lips, tongue, and the chewing muscles. Usually, only a few horses in the stable have the misfortune to become victims, but entire stables have been wiped out in a few instances. The horse with botulism

81

shows weakness and is unable to get up once he goes down. He is distressed, but not in pain. Death is caused by paralysis of the respiratory muscles, making it impossible for the victim to breathe.

Toxoids are available to immunize animals against botulism, but the control depends primarily on good management:

1/ Feed only clean, wholesome hay and grain.

2/ Avoid feeding spoiling vegetables, and *never* feed moldy or rotting hay.

3/ Clean up excess hay that horses have not eaten, especially if it has gotten wet.

4/ Protect hay from rain and snow. If it's stacked outside, be sure it is on some type of platform and is covered up.

5/ Clean out mangers and feeders regularly, especially wet debris in the bottom.

6/ Be sure the water supply is clean and fresh, and remove rotting algae from the tank.

Tail Problems

In considering health problems of the horse, we must not neglect the tail. Yes, that extremity is afflicted with problems, and we will discuss some of the more common diseases we see.

Tail rubbing. This is probably the most common complaint that the veterinarian hears concerning the tail. Pinworms are the usual cause. This parasite causes severe itching of the anus, provoking the horse to rub the base of the tail until the hair is rubbed out. Worming a horse once a year will not permanently control pinworms. In a few months the horse is usually reinfested and itching again. To control pinworms, and the even more dangerous bloodworm, it is necessary to administer medication at fairly frequent intervals.

On the same day the worm medication is administered, the entire tail area should be washed with mild soap and water. Include the area under the tail. Rinse the soap off thoroughly. This can be repeated the day after the worming as well.

We need to do this because pinworm eggs are attached to the area under the tail with a sticky cement, and it is this substance that causes the itching and

rubbing. Even if the pinworms have been killed, the itching may persist unless the hind end has been washed with soap and water.

Tail rubbing can also be caused by a dirty sheath in geldings, or by an accumulation of debris between the halves of the udder in mares. These areas should be checked and cleaned if necessary.

Seborrhea. This scaly skin disease causes loss of tail hair, flaking, dandruff, and sometimes itching. The mane can be affected, too. Shampooing these areas with a selenium sulfide shampoo (which can be prescribed by a veterinarian) is helpful. Work the medicated shampoo in well, then rinse very thoroughly. Repeat twice a week until the condition improves.

A microscopic skin parasite, *Onchoserca cervicalis*, sometimes causes a similar scaly dermatitis of the tail and/or mane. Ivermectin is effective against onchoserciasis.

Gangrene. Unfortunately, we see several cases of tail gangrene a year due to bandaging or braiding the tail too tight, cutting off the circulation. Mild cases will just lose a few patches of skin and hair, but often the entire tail below the stricture dies and must be amputated. Care must be taken not to braid tails too tightly, and not to leave tight tail wraps on too long.

Wounds. Wounds of the tail should be treated as are wounds of any other part of the body. The problem with tail wounds is that they often go unnoticed, because they are concealed with hair, until badly infected. A wound at the end of the tail is prone to bleed and ooze, and heal slowly because as the horse flips its tail, centrifugal force causes excessive bleeding. Dogs will often seize a horse's tail, causing deep puncture wounds that get infected.

Contact dermatitis. The skin of the tail—especially *under* the tail—is sensitive. A rather severe skin inflammation can be caused by any irritant. For example, the skin can be irritated in that area by diarrhea, or irritating plant chemicals in the manure. In these cases, wash the area gently and thoroughly, using Phisoderm and water. When it is dry, apply a thick layer of Desitin ointment, and repeat frequently until healed.

Soaps, fly sprays, and many other

> Unfortunately, we see several cases of tail gangrene a year due to bandaging or braiding the tail too tight, cutting off the circulation.

82

chemicals can burn the sensitive area under the tail. Various cortisone ointments help heal such skin injuries.

Melanoma. These black skin tumors are often malignant and are very common in gray horses. They may occur at any age and in any location, but they are frequently found on the tail of mature gray horses. If the tail has one or more dark lumps, melanoma must be suspected.

Fractures. A fracture of the tailbone is most common high up, close to the body. It causes a very painful swelling. The tail may hang limp and paralyzed. The veterinarian might have to X-ray the tail to confirm a fracture.

It might not be entirely pertinent to this discussion, but I will add one comment. It is my personal opinion that any operation done to inhibit the natural action of the tail in its function as a fly swatter is inhumane, and should be performed only if absolutely necessary. I make this statement fully realizing that it is the fashion in some breeds to dock the tail, or to set it, or to partially immobilize it to conceal nervous switching.

The American Quarter Horse Association, in 1986, began testing horses at shows to detect and disqualify animals with altered tails.

Skinny Horse

Inexperienced horse owners often call a veterinarian because their horses are underweight. Usually these people don't notice when the horse is 50 or so pounds lighter than he should be. Not until the horse has lost 100 or more pounds does it come to the attention of their inexperienced eyes.

Frequently they will ask the advice of a friend or neighbor who is only slightly more knowledgeable. This person will then usually inform the now worried owner that the horse probably has worms, or bad teeth, and that they had better call the vet. The veterinarian, answering a call to worm and float teeth, finds an emaciated animal. Sometimes the horse does need worming or dentistry. In fact, any horse not recently wormed usually has some parasites, and many horses have points on their teeth, or irregular edges that require rasping, but rarely are these conditions the cause

of the weight loss.

A horse's teeth have to be quite bad to make him lose weight. If the teeth are that defective, an observant owner will usually notice that the horse is having difficulty chewing. And, a well-fed horse can carry a very heavy parasite load without suffering a noticeable weight loss. Most well-fed horses will stay fat, even if loaded with worms. They might look fairly healthy, but also have a dull hair coat, and have a wormy look to an experienced horseman, but they can remain in good flesh.

The fact is that most of the skinny horses I see in my practice are simply not being fed enough. A lot of horse owners feed a flake of hay twice a day and expect the horse to stay fat. If he loses weight, they blame his teeth, or his worms. What is a flake of hay? It will vary in weight and consistency. What kind of hay is it? How good is it? How old is it? When was it cut? How well was it cured? What kind of a hay baler baled it? In other words, is it a good-quality thick flake, or a poor-quality thin flake?

A horse ration should be determined in pounds, not in flakes. Most mature horses require 1½ to 2 pounds of dry feed, per 100 pounds of body weight daily. So, a 1,000-pound horse will require 15 to 20 pounds of hay a day. If he is fed two flakes weighing six pounds each, he is going to be a skinny horse in a couple of months.

If a horse is working fairly hard, or is a hard keeper, it might be impossible to keep him in proper condition without feeding grain. I often ask owners who are concerned about their horse's underweight condition why they aren't feeding

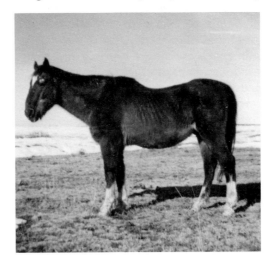

some grain. The answers vary:

"He doesn't need grain. I only ride three hours a day."

"He gets too high and silly on grain. I can't control him."

"My other horse stays fat on hay alone."

"Grain is too expensive. I'm saving my money for a new horse." (And you'll need one, too, because this horse is starving to death.)

I repeat: Most skinny horses are simply not getting enough to eat. Their bodies are burning more calories than they are consuming. Regular worming and dentistry are important, but are no substitute for a proper diet. The same is true of vitamins. They are fine for your horse, but they won't add weight when calories are what he needs. A skinny horse needs lots of food, regardless of what else is done. Feed him plenty of hay. Also feed a couple of pounds of grain a day, and more if he is working daily. Don't eliminate exercise. Continue moderate exercise, but increase his calorie intake.

When two or more horses are quartered together, it is not unusual to see one lose weight. Again, the owner may conclude that the thin horse has more worms or worse teeth than the fatter horse. But usually the explanation is that the fatter horse dominates the thin horse and eats his fill, while the skinny one gets the leftovers. Or, sometimes, the faster eater gets a sufficient amount, and the slow eater gradually starves.

If a properly fed horse loses weight, even with good dental care and parasite control, a thorough physical examination is called for. I examine such a horse, and take laboratory tests to rule out metabolic problems or a hidden disease. The horse might have liver disease, anemia, diabetes, cancer, chronic infection, or any number of other problems that cause weight loss. Diseases of the pituitary gland, the adrenal glands, the thyroid, the kidney, the heart, or the intestine can all cause weight loss. Keep in mind, however, that these are all relatively infrequent. An empty belly explains most skinny horses.

On a skinny-horse call, I check the stable to see if there is any feed left over. Most of the time, the horse has cleaned up every morsel and is eating the barn, the fences, and the corral. I'll usually ask the owner to feed the horse his regular ration so I can see exactly how much is fed. On one call, a 13-year-old boy fed two big flakes of hay. I asked in surprise, "Do you feed that twice a day?"

"No," he said. "I feed that every other day. In between, I give him a can of grain."

Finally, we must realize that some horses, like some people, are just naturally lean no matter how much they eat. Such individuals, however, even though thin, have a healthy, vigorous look about them. In the case of show horses with such a metabolism, the owner will often feed concentrates to a hazardous extreme and still not get the horse as plump as he'd like. Overfeeding grain is an invitation to founder or azoturia. Instead, try feeding this kind of horse a cup or two of corn oil daily. I have recommended this for many years. The oil is very high in calories, palatable to the horse, and does not seem to cause digestive problems or cause founder or azoturia. As a bonus, it helps to put a sheen on the coat.

Obesity

It has been said that overeating is the greatest single health hazard in the United States today. A great number of human diseases may be blamed wholly or partially on overeating. To combat this problem, health experts have long campaigned for proper nutrition, and as a result we hear and read about this diet and that.

There are banana diets and fruit juice diets, canned diets, and drinking man's diets, high fat diets and low calorie diets, low fat diets and high protein diets, sensible diets and non-sensical diets. However, the sum total of all this furor is this: Obesity is undesirable. It is detrimental to good health.

If this be true in man, why not in beast? Why is it that so many horse show judges, particularly in the stock horse breeds (and a stock horse is supposed to be an athlete) will consistently favor the fat—yes, I said *fat*—horse over an equally good horse in *lean, good shape?* Are we raising our horses for meat? Is the dog food factory the real goal in raising horses? When we say "stock horse," do we mean a horse that *works* stock, or a horse that *is* stock?

Should we start raising beef and dairy-type horses, and look forward to such future delicacies in the frozen food department as "Appaloosa round steak" and "fermented mare's milk?" Will there eventually be lard-type horses and bacon-type horses? We've already got the lard-type horse; you can see him in any western halter class. We've got the bacon-type too; you can see him at any race track, rodeo arena, or round-up remuda.

Obesity is a disease in horses just as it is in man. To me, as a veterinarian, it is unsightly and unhealthy. Yet, as a horse breeder, I am well aware of the pressure I am under to overfeed my stock in order to place high in halter classes. I place the blame on the judges and on the breed associations. A strong educational campaign must be waged to stipulate that judges *mark down* fat horses in conformation classes. As soon as fat horses start to fail in the shows, then the people who own and show good horses are going to start feeding correctly and our horses will enjoy better health.

So what's wrong with fat horses?

1/ Fat horses cannot be as agile as lean horses (I said "lean," not underweight). Did you ever see a fat horse at the race track? Of course not! They're lean and hard. They are "in shape." And they look great, don't they?

2/ Excessive weight puts a strain on the musculoskeletal system of young growing horses. Bones, joints, tendons, and ligaments are all more susceptible to injury when the animal is packing extra weight, especially when these structures are still tender and immature.

3/ Obesity in broodmares and stallions interferes with fertility. Fat breeding animals are often known to be poor breeders.

4/ Selection of fat-prone individuals as winning types is detrimental to any breed. Such individuals aren't likely to perform well or breed well. One of the differences between "halter-type" and "using-type" stock horses is the fat-prone metabolism in the halter type. The horse is a *using* animal; and the type that performs well on the track or in the arena is the type that should win at halter.

5/ Fat horses are prone to founder.

This can be a cause or an effect. Some horses are fed so much grain in order to get them in show shape that they founder. In others, the body weight is so excessive that they will "road founder" from excessive concussion when used hard.

6/ Fat-type horses are sometimes hypothyroid. Such thyroid-deficient animals are excessively easy keepers, prone to founder, poor breeders, and fat. Some judges actually place the hypothyroid-type mare on top of the halter class.

7/ "Pushing the feed" to show horses can and does produce some very serious metabolic disorders. Azoturia is an example. A more common problem occurs in the fat, growing foal fed excessive quantities of grain.

Grain contains great quantities of several compounds and elements such as phytic acid, which interferes with the absorption of calcium. As a result, a calcium deficiency occurs in the body, despite the presence of adequate quantities of calcium in the ration, in the form of milk, bone meal, alfalfa, or mineral supplements. Since it is imperative that the calcium level of the blood be maintained in order for life to go on, the bones are robbed of calcium. Consequently, many fat, heavily grained colts have bone disease.

Marginal cases may manifest no obvious abnormality, but the damage is there, perhaps to show up later in life by premature and disabling lameness. In many other cases, the damage is quite obvious to the observer. Such colts may have enlarged knobby joints, tenderness, vague lameness, and swelling of the limbs. When you combine soft bone with excessive weight, permanent damage follows.

Remember that the calcium deficiency in these animals *cannot* be corrected by feeding calcium. Their problem is that they cannot *absorb* the calcium already passing through their digestive tract. In order for them to absorb it, the grain ration must be drastically reduced.

This fact is little known in the horse world, and, in my opinion, is the single greatest reason why horse show judges should be prejudiced against fat colts. There is irrefutable scientific evidence that excessive graining does interfere with normal bone metabolism.

8/ As every showman knows, you can conceal a lot of defects with fat. A horse with a lot of minor conformation faults can, when fat, present a deceptive impression of smoothness. This may explain why a breeder may want a fat horse, but how in the world can it explain a judge placing such a horse high in a halter class?

I am reminded of the plump, middle-aged lady who said, "I'm glad I'm overweight because it fills my face out and I don't have any wrinkles." To this her lean companion commented, "That's true, honey, but don't forget that the wrinkles are there anyway. They just don't show."

Really, all we have to do is apply common sense to nutrition. There isn't a lot we know about equine nutrition, although research is being done. Meanwhile, let's use our heads. Nature intended the horse to nurse as a foal, and to eat grass. In addition, he exercised by running free in the sunshine on open plains.

Keeping a yearling in a box stall with a blanket on and cramming him full of all the grain he can hold, plus seven different supplements and conditioners is a long way from the way his mustang ancestor lived.

Let's apply common sense—or should we call it horse sense—in raising horses. They need exercise and sunshine, clean water and salt, and a diet of good hay (including at least a third alfalfa or other legume hay) or good green pasture; plus enough grass seed (grain) to keep them in good flesh or compensate for the calories burned up by training or work. To make sure that no deficiencies exist, select a complete balanced vitamin-mineral supplement manufactured by a reputable company and then—for gosh sakes—don't try to improve the product they worked so hard to perfect by adding your own little secret ingredients.

Remember the man whose veterinarian told him to give the sick horse enough medicated powder to cover a dime? He didn't have a dime so he used ten pennies. As he buried the horse he observed, "Just because a little bit is good, that doesn't mean a whole lot is better."

Remember that no one supplement can supply the needs of every geographi-cal area. Some areas, even certain farms, have special mineral and vitamin deficiencies or imbalances, depending on soil conditions, fertilization programs, type of forage available, and so on. Consult your local veterinarian, state agricultural college, county agent, or some other reliable authority for his advice as to feeding your horses. And I said *feeding*—not *overfeeding*.

Before concluding, I would like to add that there are people who do not feed their horses enough. Sometimes this is through lack of proper knowledge, sometimes it's through neglect, and sometimes it is intentional. As an example of the latter: horse trainers who deliberately underfeed their horses so they will be lethargic in the show ring.

Underfeeding, to an extreme, is just as bad as overfeeding.

Choke

In horses, choke is a frightening, and often misunderstood phenomenon. In humans, the term "choke" usually refers to an obstruction of the airway, usually with a chunk of food such as a piece of meat. It is a dire emergency because the offending object has been inhaled into the larynx (the voice box or opening into the windpipe). The patient cannot get air, and without air we die rather quickly. Sometimes the foreign body is inhaled right down into the windpipe.

Such a choke, in humans, is a desperately serious situation, and I hope that all of us are familiar with the Heimlich maneuver, wherein the diaphragm is suddenly and forcefully compressed. This maneuver will, hopefully, expel the foreign body, and the patient is saved.

In horses, choke is also caused by a bolus (lump) of food, but it doesn't go down into the windpipe, causing an obstruction to breathing. Instead, the offending mass sticks in the esophagus, also called the gullet, or the food pipe. This is very uncomfortable, and it causes a lot of distressing symptoms, but it is not immediately dangerous. It is never immediately life-threatening.

The horse choking due to an obstructed esophagus has no problem breathing. He can't eat anything. He can't drink. He is uncomfortable and he may be frightened. Large quantities of saliva, usually stained green from feed, come flowing and bubbling out of his mouth and from his nostrils, but he *can* breathe.

So, when a horse chokes, don't panic. Call the vet, but keep cool. A horse can have his esophagus obstructed all day, or even several days, and still recover.

Of course, the obstruction *must* be relieved. The horse cannot eat or drink as long as the choke is present. Moreover, if the mass in the esophagus stays there, it will eventually cause erosion and rupture of the esophagus. This is fatal, but it takes a long time.

Choke in horses is usually due to greedy feeding, and inadequately chewing. Pellets cause choke more often than does hay, but that doesn't mean that pellets often cause choke.

We have thousands of our patients on pelleted feed, but we only see a few cases of choke a year. Moreover, I find pellet chokes easier to treat than hay chokes because pellets disintegrate when moistened. Horses that habitually gobble pellets too fast can be slowed down by putting large round stones in the manger, about the size of a loaf of bread.

I don't think I have ever seen a horse choke on chopped hay, or on cubed hay. The most difficult chokes to relieve are those caused by long-stemmed, coarse hay. Horses sometimes choke on corncobs, or on apples or carrots. Apples and carrots can be sliced to lessen the likelihood of choke.

The choke can occur anywhere along the course of the esophagus, between the throat and the stomach, but the most frequent locations seem to be the throat, in the first few inches of the esophagus (and these are difficult to relieve), the thoracic inlet (at the base of the neck), and over the heart, within the chest.

Some chokes will relieve themselves, but one must never count on this. Occasionally, tranquilizing a horse will allow him to swallow the choking object, probably by causing simple relaxation.

Acupuncture has helped horses with choke. The needle is inserted in an anatomical point below the ear. Most chokes are relieved when the veterinarian passes a stomach tube through the horse's nostril, down the esophagus, to the obstruction, and then, with the aid of lubricants, pushes the foreign body down into the stomach.

But sometimes, the object cannot be moved. There are drugs that can relax the esophagus and stimulate swallowing. Sometimes we have to give up and try again a few hours later. As a last resort, surgery may have to be employed, but I have never found this necessary.

It is important to try to relieve the problem before the lining of the esophagus is damaged, because scar tissue can cause a stricture or narrowing of the esophagus, with permanent recurring problems.

After recovering from a choke, a horse should be fed tiny, moist meals until the swelling of the esophagus lining is gone, or he may choke again. This may take several days.

Tics and Vices

A tic (not to be confused with tick, a tiny parasite) is a habitually repeated, purposeless movement, usually involving a particular muscle group. Tics are also known as habit spasms, mimic spasms; some people call them twitches. In people, tics are most common around the head and neck. People with nervous tics blink, nod, shrug, move their jaws, clench their teeth, purse their lips, wink, clear their throat, swallow, cough, or shake their head.

True tics can be controlled by the patient, at least for a while, and they disappear during sleep. Excitement, emotional stress, and fatigue will usually increase the tic. In other words, a tic is usually a nervous habit. Occasionally, a tic can be caused by brain damage.

Do tics occur in horses? Yes, they do. Yet, I have never seen a tic described in any book about horses I have ever read. Most horse books talk about vices, but to me there is a distinct difference between a tic and a vice, although some vices, as I shall point out, may actually be tics.

A tic is quick, repetitive, and involves a limited muscle group. Most vices, on the other hand, are prolonged bad habits and completely under the control of the horse.

Before I describe some tics in horses, let me give examples of vices first. Vices are undesirable bad habits in the horse and are usually divided into three types.

Most horse books talk about vices, but to me there is a distinct difference between a tic and a vice, although some vices, as I shall point out, may actually be tics.

I'll give examples of each.

STABLE VICES

Kicking at passing horses or people.
Pulling back when tied.
Tearing up blankets.
Wood chewing.
Manure eating.
Pawing.
Biting or charging passers-by.

GENERAL VICES

Refusing to be caught.
Rearing while being cinched.
Kicking, striking, biting, or charging.
Pulling back.
Shying with head and being difficult to bridle.

VICES WHEN MOUNTED

Rearing.
Bucking.
Whirling and shying.
Running away.
Rolling.
Jigging.
Balking.
Boring (lowering the head and ignoring the bit).
Grazing while mounted.
Fighting other horses.
Nickering and whinnying.

All of the vices I have described are certainly bad habits. Most are the result of training errors. Most are correctable by skilled, persistent, and consistent trainers.

Now let's describe some tics.

I am often asked to see a horse that snaps his head as if an insect were going up his nose. The owner is often positive that bees or flies or tiny gnats are to blame. I sometimes have a hard time convincing him that no insects are involved. I point out that the habit is not present when the horse is asleep or completely relaxed and alone in the stall or corral. I remind him that none of the other horses are doing this head jerking. (Remember that all horses will do this at the times when bot and nose flies are active.) Most important, I show him that the horse makes his sudden head motions only when he is under pressure (being worked). Despite my efforts, many owners remain convinced that invisible bugs are flying up the horse's nose, and smear the nose with all kinds of concoctions to keep the bugs away. This sudden snap of the head, frequently repeated, is a common tic in horses.

Another common tic is the "bug in the ear" syndrome. I have heard cowboys refer to it as "sour ear." This horse is often ear-shy but not necessarily so. (An ear-shy horse has a vice in which it will not allow one or both ears to be touched.) The horse with an ear tic acts like something is in his ear; he lowers the ear, shakes his head, nods his head, etc. The owner usually decides the horse has an ear tick.

Wait! This is confusing! Let's distinguish between an ear tic (a habit) and an ear tick (a parasite bug that lives in the ear). A horse with an ear *tic* will only go into his act when bridled and worked.

A horse with ear *ticks* will show discomfort when at rest in the stall or pasture.

I do believe that many *tics* start with *ticks*, and then become habitual. Examination of the ear by a veterinarian, and observation of the behavior pattern will help differentiate tic from tick.

I mentioned earlier that there are vices that may actually be tics. Perhaps this kind of tic starts as a controllable vice, and later develops into an uncontrollable tic. Here are a few common examples:

1/ Cribbing, in which the horse seizes a post or rail with his teeth, arches his neck, grunts, and swallows air.

2/ Windsucking is similar to cribbing except that the horse doesn't have to grab something with his teeth.

3/ Weaving is a common habit in nervous horses confined to stalls. The weaver rhythmically swings his head and sways from side to side in the stall.

4/ Stall walking is similar to weaving except that instead of just moving the fore half of the body, the horse nervously circles the stall, or paces back and forth like many caged zoo animals do.

5/ Tail switching is often seen in show horses undergoing pressure training. It can become such a persistent vice that it is properly called a tic.

Tics and vices both result from mental and environmental stresses. These include:

1/ A nervous temperament combined with high-energy diets.

2/ Confinement. A horse's heritage is to roam open plains, not be locked up in small stalls or paddocks.

3/ Errors in handling, especially with initial experiences such as the first shoeing, first saddling, first trailering, first clipping, or first doctoring.

4/ Too much training pressure. Each horse differs in intelligence, flightiness, submissiveness, ability to learn, and ability to retain. Horses' aptitudes vary, as do their athletic abilities. The trainer must therefore vary his or her technique, pace, attitude, and style to avoid excessive pressure on the horse's nervous system. Professional trainers sometimes subject their horses to more pressure than they can endure. In other cases, the trainer does a fine job, but the owner rides the horse improperly, causing the horse to suffer confusion and nervousness. When a horse starts to tic, that horse is undergoing emotional stress and an objective analysis of its cause should be made. The horse may need less food and less schooling, and more room and more cross-country riding.

Tongue Injuries

If you look in a lot of horses' mouths, you will see a lot of mutilated and deformed tongues. Most often, the tongue has been partially cut through in its middle portion, and has healed leaving a constricted portion. Once in a while, you'll find a horse with part of his tongue missing.

These injuries are most frequently caused by a bit. Because the bit fits over the tongue, it can damage that organ if sudden, severe pressure is applied to the bit. This can occur when a horse steps on the reins, or when a horse suddenly pulls back when tied by the reins. Less often, it can be caused by a strong, crude rider, hauling back sharply on the reins.

Any kind of bit can cut the tongue, but some kinds of mouthpieces are obviously more traumatic than others, For example, a rubber snaffle is very unlikely to cut the tongue, whereas a twisted wire mouthpiece could do so rather easily.

The tongue is a vascular organ with a very rich blood supply. Even a small wound will produce a large amount of blood, and a larger wound will bleed in such quantity that it often panics the owner. Remember that a horse has a lot of blood, and that horse blood clots

rather slowly. So don't get excited if you see a wound of this kind. I have never seen a horse bleed to death from a tongue wound, even when the tongue was badly cut or actually severed.

Smaller wounds of the tongue will heal with virtually no treatment, and with rare complications, although the usual precautions against tetanus and infection should be taken.

Severe lacerations will require surgical repair if mutilation is to be prevented. Repairing a major tongue wound is no easy task for the veterinary surgeon. The wound is in a cramped place, which makes access difficult, and the suturing of an active, moving muscular organ like the tongue requires very exacting surgical technique if success is to be expected. Even utilizing general anesthesia and good surgery, failures will occur.

Fortunately, horses can function quite well with a mutilated tongue, and even without a tongue. Horses do not use the tongue to pull grass to them as do cattle; horses use their lips. They do not use the tongue to drink as dogs and cats do. A horse with a deformed or missing tongue functions quite well.

There are other ways in which horses can suffer tongue injuries. In my part of the country (southern California), all of the native grasses have penetrating awns on their seeds. These seeds are collectively known as foxtails. Masses of these

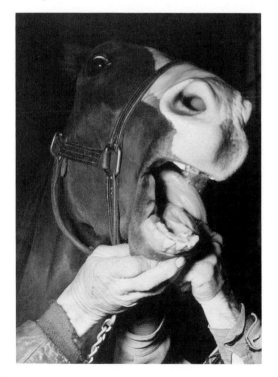

foxtails often embed in the mouth or under the tongue, causing drooling, foul odor, and ulcerated sores.

Licking metal in very cold weather can damage the tongue. Horsemen should remember this before putting a cold bit in the horse's mouth, or feeding grain in a metal container in frigid weather.

Licking corrosive substances can burn the mouth and tongue. Such substances include paints, creosote, lye, and slaked lime.

The tongue can also be cut if a horse licks broken glass. I saw this happen once when a jar of honey fell off a shelf and broke.

It's not unusual for a horse to bite his own tongue hard enough to cause bleeding, especially in a fall.

In summary, tongue injuries are fairly frequent in equine practice. They bleed profusely, but they heal well and rarely handicap the horse.

Chronic Equine Abscesses

During the late 1950s, a problem appeared in California horses that has plagued them ever since. The problem was an outbreak of abscesses, usually localized in the chest muscles, caused by a bacteria called *Corynebacterium pseudotuberculosis.* The disease, usually simply called chest abscess, has also been called dryland distemper, dryland strangles, false distemper, pigeon fever, and breastbone fever. Since this disease is in no way related to distemper or strangles, the most appropriate name is chest abscess.

Affected horses usually show a diffuse, painful swelling of the pectoral muscles, with much surrounding edema and inflammation. In some cases the abscess involves the sheath of the gelding, the udder of the mare, or the belly wall. But most involve the lower body wall from the chest to the groin. There may be one or several abscesses, appearing simultaneously or following one another. Often the infection is mixed— that is, other bacteria are found in the abscess. Also, the same horse may be affected year after year.

After a few weeks, the abscesses rupture and drain, and with the exception of very rare fatalities due to internal abscesses, the horse recovers completely. The course of the disease may be hastened by hot packing or poulticing the abscess area, and by surgically draining the abscess after it is ripe (comes to a head).

There are many cases in California every year, and the disease is now being seen all over the country. Some years there are epidemics involving scores of horses, but the abscesses do not seem to be directly contagious from horse to horse. Despite intensive studies, the means of transmission has not been found. It is suspected, however, that the infection is carried by flies or by migrating parasitic larvae. There are no *known* means of either prevention or cure.

Systematic use of antibiotics will ordinarily fail to stop the abscesses, and will, in fact, prolong the course of the disease. But *some* cases require antibiotics, if the infection becomes generalized. Since the mortality rate is low, the disease is mostly a nuisance that only time, patience, and normal body defenses will heal.

Cribbing

Cribbing is one of the most senseless, costly, and annoying vices that horses are subject to. The habit is also known as crib biting and wind sucking. A crib is an old name for what we now call a manger, hence the term cribbing, but a horse may crib on a fence, water trough, barn door, or almost any other projection at the proper height, as well as on a manger.

When a horse cribs he forcibly swallows large gulps of air. In order to accomplish this he seizes an object with his teeth, flexes his neck sharply, pulls upward, and sucks in a gulp of air with an audible grunt. The habit is so idiotic and purposeless, and does so much damage to the horse, that the owner soon finds himself in a duel trying to outwit the horse.

Do not confuse ordinary wood chewing with cribbing. Wood chewing can be a troublesome vice, but unless it is accompanied by the bent neck and the air swallowing, it should not be called cribbing. However, it is possible for wood chewing to develop into true cribbing, so corrective measure should be taken to stop ordinary wood chewing.

It is difficult for horses to belch up gas. Therefore, the continuous swallowing of air leads to chronic inflammation of the stomach or intestines. Such a horse loses condition and stamina. He grows unthrifty in appearance, and much of his food is poorly digested. In a really bad cribber the incisor teeth become bevelled and worn. This, incidentally, is one way to spot a cribber when buying a horse. The worst cribbers wear their incisor teeth to the gum, and become so emaciated that, unless corrective measures are taken, their very life is in danger. I recall one fine Quarter Horse mare that, due to the owner's indifference, actually cribbed herself to death from malnutrition. Most cases, of course, aren't nearly this severe, but all cribbers suffer for their habit.

What makes a horse crib? Horsemen have wondered about this for centuries. Many years ago it was thought to be caused by gas in the stomach. Now we know that the gas is the *result*, not the *cause* of cribbing. Another old theory was that the teeth were too long, and to stop the cribbing the owner would cut or file the incisor teeth down. This did, indeed, stop the cribbing for a while, but only because of the pain involved. The modern concept is that cribbing is a vice of psychological origin. I suppose it might be compared to nail biting in humans, or knuckle cracking, or similar habits. Factors involved in cribbing are boredom, confinement in too-close quarters, nutritional deficiencies, and learning it from another horse.

However, there must also be a basic predisposition to the vice. The problem is worse in Thoroughbreds, probably because the colts are in high condition and raring to go, and often confined to a lonely stall. In other words, we have an individual full of youthful energy, and nothing to do. So he cribs, or weaves, or walks the stall, or adopts some other vice. Don't human youngsters make a good analogy? If every American teenager played a fast game of basketball, or spent a few hours on horseback every day, there would be less juvenile delinquency.

What can be done to help a cribber? To actually *remove* the desire to crib from his mind is almost impossible. But a great variety of methods have been devised to *control* the habit. Years ago these included such barbaric devices as wedges driven between the teeth, and metal plates bolted between them. If such methods worked, it was only because cribbing became too painful for the horse to endure.

A more acceptable method is the use of a cribbing strap. This consists of a heavy strap, 3 or 3½ inches wide, buckled snugly (not too snug) around the throat. When he flexes his neck to crib, the strap cuts off his wind. The cribbing strap works well on mild cases. A confirmed addict needs stronger treatment. The cribbing strap may be embellished with a row of seven or eight sharp tacks on the area under the throat. The strap is adjusted so that the tacks never touch the skin unless the horse arches his neck to crib.

A variety of commercial cribbing straps have been designed, with prongs and even electric shockers to punish the horse when he tries to crib.

Fences and other objects cribbed on may be painted with tabasco sauce, or other unpalatable substances. Or they may be electrically wired. For intractable cases a surgical cribbing operation may be performed on the neck to limit the action of the muscles used in cribbing. The operation works well, but is somewhat disfiguring.

In the case of a colt just starting to crib, be sure he has plenty of room to exercise, and can see other horses, people, automobile traffic, etc., to distract him. A goat or burro for company might help. Get him away from any other horses that crib.

Have a veterinarian experienced in equine practice check his diet and prescribe a vitamin supplement. Be sure he is free of worms. A little steamed bone meal on grain has been reported to be effective in these early cases. I would recommend that in such a case, the use of pelleted feeds be avoided. Chewing on hay or pasture will keep the colt more occupied. While these environmental changes are being created, the colt may be kept lightly tranquilized.

For the confirmed cribber, there is no such thing as a sure cure. The worst cases will even crib on their own lower

91

lip. But, for *nearly* all cases, the following suggestions will stop cribbing:

Build a corral of steel fence posts. Wire it with two rows of electrically charged wire. Have the top wire insulators set right at the top of the posts.

For a shelter build a shed with its supporting walls outside the electric fence, and with its roof overhanging and projecting into the corral. A horse will not crib on anything below his knees, so provide a metal water trough and a masonry manger built low at ground level. Provide salt and bone meal in granular form, in similar low containers. In such a corral, an unthrifty cribber will quickly gain weight and vigor.

General First Aid

Nature intended the horse to run loose out on the open plains. Domestication, with its barbed wire, broken glass, nails, splinters, and chafing saddles, has provided the horse a multitude of opportunities for a wide variety of injuries.

When we think of wounds in horses, it is vital that we also think of tetanus. Horses are very susceptible to this dread infection and, unfortunately, the tetanus germ is a common inhabitant of the horse's own intestinal tract. The tetanus germ cannot grow in the presence of air, so any wound deep enough to exclude air is a potential site for a tetanus infection. Most dangerous of all are puncture wounds, such as nail punctures, splinters, bullet wounds, and "quicking" during horseshoeing.

The best method of preventing tetanus is to be sure that your horse is vaccinated with tetanus toxoid and boostered annually. For horses that have never been vaccinated against tetanus, or for which the history is unknown, an injection of tetanus antitoxin will confer temporary, but effective immunity.

But don't confuse the two. Tetanus toxoid is a vaccine used *before* the horse suffers a wound. It causes the horse to make its own antibodies against the tetanus toxin. Tetanus antitoxin is made from the blood serum of immunized horses. It simply *loans* antibodies to the horse to whom it is given, which will protect it for a week or two.

Severe lacerations will require professional attention. Such wounds can often be sutured, which will result in quicker healing and less scar tissue. Avoid home treatment of such wounds if you are calling a veterinarian. Improper treatment or delay may interfere with his surgical repair.

Bleeding wounds are best controlled with direct pressure. Apply a thick bandage to the wound with gentle pressure and leave it there. Even if the bandage soaks through, it will serve as a matrix to help the bleeding to stop by forming a blood clot. Horses have a *lot* of blood, so don't panic if the wound bleeds. We take a full gallon of blood from a horse for a transfusion, and that amount doesn't even faze him. Also, horse blood clots slowly, so don't be alarmed if bleeding doesn't stop for 15 or 20 minutes.

If a major artery is cut—and I mean a major artery, not a little one—you will see a serious hemorrhage that spurts with each heartbeat. Such bleeding must be controlled, and under those circumstances, a tourniquet may be used. Of course, a tourniquet can only be used if the bleeding is from a wound in a limb, and the tourniquet must be applied *above* the wound to shut off the blood supply coming from the heart. If a veterinarian cannot see the horse quickly, don't forget to loosen the tourniquet for half a minute every half-hour to permit some circulation into the limb.

What about the minor cuts horses are forever getting? Clean with a gentle antiseptic or sterile saline solution. Your veterinarian will suggest his favorite medication. The important things to remember are to avoid strong, burning, irritating medicines, and to avoid the great temptation to overtreat. Frequent applications of a half-dozen salves plus sheep dip and bacon grease will only retard healing and result in a nastier scar.

One of the commonest complications of horse wounds is excessive granulation or proud flesh. Proud flesh is caused by irritating medication, oils and greases, and constant movement, as in the hock or pastern region. Some wounds would actually heal better if left untreated than they do after being repeatedly painted with some of the junk on the stable shelf. Clean the wound. Apply a gentle antiseptic. Then leave it alone.

During fly season, a repellent dressing may be necessary. Once again, consult your veterinarian. In this age of wonder drugs, it is inexcusable to pour sheep dip or axle grease into a wound.

Cinch and saddle sores shouldn't occur if your equipment is clean and fits properly. Nevertheless, they will happen. The best treatment is rest until healed, but if you must ride with a sore, here are some suggestions. For a cinch sore, use a double-rigged saddle with a breast collar. Tighten your flank cinch a little bit. Now you can loosen your front cinch. Cover the cinch over the sore with a sheepskin pad. Powder generously with a mixture of 90 percent talcum powder (or you can use baby powder), 10 percent boric acid, and 10 percent zinc oxide. This lubricating powder is fine for cinch and saddle sores. Bathe sore backs with cool water. Cut a hole in a felt saddle pad over the sore. Powder generously. A commercial gall lotion will help dry the moist, weeping sore.

Nowadays, we fight infections from the inside; that is, with antibiotics and sulfonamides.

To sum up, when your horse is wounded, consider tetanus, avoid overtreatment, keep the flies away, and give nature a chance. Veterinary advice is as close as your telephone.

Best of all, try to prevent wounds by exercising care and common sense; watch where you ride, avoid loose barbed wire, pull that rusty nail sticking out of the stall partition, brush his back before saddling, wash that saddle blanket, and, on a long ride, get off once in a while, raise the saddle skirts, and let his back cool a bit.

First-Aid Kit

Every horseman should keep a few items in a portable kit that serves as a first-aid kit for horses. This kit and its contents can provide certain necessary items, on hand immediately, should you need them for treating the horse yourself or in the event that your veterinarian prescribes their use before his arrival. I recommend that the kit include the following items:

1/ A box of Epsom salts, to be used as directed by a veterinarian.

2/ Hydrogen peroxide, for cleansing

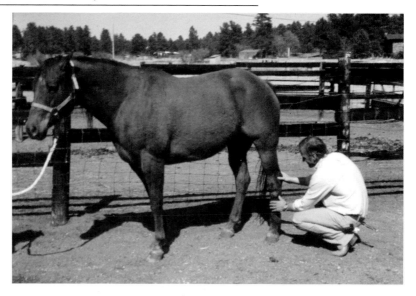

fresh wounds.

3/ A sulfonamide or antibiotic powder for dusting fresh wounds after cleansing, or you can use nitrofurazone cream or liquid if you prefer.

4/ Povidol iodine solution ("tamed" iodine or betadine). It can be used to treat thrush, nail punctures of the foot, and ringworm. Diluted with water (1:4), it can also be used to irrigate wounds.

5/ A fly repellent wound dressing. Ask your veterinarian to prescribe one for minor wounds. There are several products available.

6/ A fly repellent that can be used close to the eyes. One of the mosquito repellent sticks used by fishermen and campers is suitable, but there are products available in tack shops made specifically for horses.

7/ A pint of rubbing alcohol.

8/ A rectal veterinary thermometer. (In hot weather, protect the thermometer from breaking by keeping it in a cooler or in your pocket.)

9/ A supply of dressings, including cotton, sterile gauze pads, a thick absorbent wound dressing, bandages, adhesive tape, and elastic bandage.

Other useful first-aid necessities will be found in any well-equipped stable. These include a hoof pick, hoof knife, a can of hoof dressing, a twitch, a pair of bandage scissors, and a pair of fencing pliers (to free a horse caught in wire).

You'll notice that this kit is simple and doesn't contain a lot of fancy remedies. What it does contain, however, is adequate to take care of the ordinary mishaps.

Here are a few first-aid reminders:

1/ *Colic*—Walk the horse. Do not feed. Call the veterinarian immediately.

2/ *Azoturia*—Do not move the horse. Call the veterinarian immediately.

3/ *Minor wounds*—Clean with peroxide or betadine or saline solution. Dust with a wound powder. Apply a fly repellent dressing around the wound if necessary. Do not overtreat.

4/ *Major wounds*—If bleeding badly, apply a pressure dressing over the wound. Do not apply wound lotions, smears, or iodine. They might interfere with the veterinarian's job when he arrives.

5/ *Acute fresh bruises, strains, swellings*—Apply cold packs. Do not use liniments on such injuries when they are fresh.

6/ *Fractures, trailer accident injuries, etc.*—Quietly free the horse. Try to calm him down. Apply pressure to severely bleeding wounds, and padded splints to any broken legs. *Do not* excite the horse. Call the veterinarian.

7/ *Founder*—Call the veterinarian at once. If the founder is due to gorging on grain, do not offer food or water.

8/ *Heat stroke*—Move the horse out of the sun. If his temperature is over 103°F, bathe him with cool water.

For pain, if veterinary drugs are not available, a horse can be given regular 15-grain human aspirin tablets. A full-sized horse will require 10 to 15 tablets, depending on his size.

Bandaging

The subject of bandaging, even if confined to the legs, is so complex and varied that I decided to show just a few of the more difficult leg bandages, for the areas where horse owners seem to get in trouble the most. In this series I will show methods of bandaging the knee (carpus), hock, and two methods of bandaging the lower leg. Although leg bandages are often used for support and for protection in horses, the ones I have selected are with injuries in mind. These are bandages that serve to cover wounds (whether sutured or not), contusions, abrasions, and also bruised or swollen areas where it is desirable to apply some sort of poultice, and keep it in contact with the leg.

BANDAGE SUPPLIES

Although I am not one to encourage elaborate stable or trail first-aid kits filled with all sorts of elaborate medications, I do think that the horse owner needs a variety of bandaging and dressing materials on hand for the inevitable injuries that occur, especially to the legs. The following list of supplies includes the ones that I use most frequently. They are available from pharmacies, veterinarians, surgical or physicians' supply houses, and some of them can be found in tack shops.

1/ Wound coverings:

a/ Four-inch gauze sponges are good. Individual sterile-wrapped sponges are available, or they can be purchased in larger packets.

b/ Telsa bandages are nice because they are sterile and because they don't stick to the wound.

2/ Roller gauze bandage: For horses, the four-inch width serves all needs, and I like the elastic "cling" gauze.

3/ Absorbent cotton: Have several rolls on hand.

4/ Elastic bandages, three- or four-inch widths:

a/ Ace elastic bandages.

b/ Vetrap, an excellent paper product, available in colors. It sticks to itself and can be molded and pressed after application into a cast-like shell.

c/ Elastic adhesive bandage: In my opinion, the greatest bandage ever manufactured for use on the horse. Two brand names are Elastikon and Elastoplast.

5/ Unna's Boot (Gelocast): A cloth bandage impregnated with zinc oxide and gelatin, it was designed for use in human leg ulcers. However, it has become a very popular leg bandage for horses. Brand names include Gelocast (which my clients also call "jellycast" or "Jello-cast"), and Linicast.

This bandage is a favorite of mine, but there is a trick to applying it and I do not recommend it for the novice because, if done improperly, serious leg damage can result. This bandage is best prescribed by a veterinarian and if he or she wants you to apply it, ask for a demonstration.

6/ A roll of plastic food wrapping like SaranWrap or GladWrap. Useful when applying an "occlusive bandage." For example, use it to cover nitrofurazone

(Furacin) ointment to "sweat" a swollen limb, or use it to cover Icthammol or Numotizine ointment when poulticing an infected limb. Change dressing daily.

There are two more types of bandage that I think horsemen should be aware of.

The first is the U.S. Army Field Bandage. In military surplus stores, one can often find U.S. Army Type One Field Bandages, which are very convenient for bandaging horses' legs. The large, thick, absorbent bandage comes wrapped in a sterile package, also containing two rolls of four-inch cling-type gauze bandage and a package of large safety pins. They make a handy item to take along on trail rides, or to stow in the tack box of a horse trailer. The pictures here show how the bandage can be used on legs. Obviously, the bandage can also be used to cover wounds elsewhere on the body, or if a human is injured.

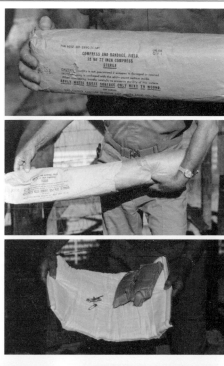

1A—The packaged field bandage.

2A—Removing the bandage from its sterile wrapper.

3A—Inside the bandage are two sterile wrapped rolls of gauze and safety pins.

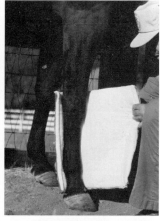

4A—The opened bandage is just the right size to wrap around the lower leg of a horse.

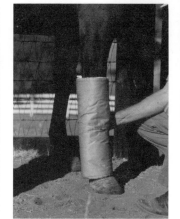

5A—The bandage snugly wrapped around the leg.

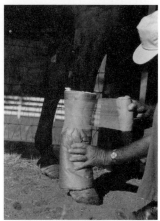

6A—Next, using the four-inch roller gauze bandage, snugly wrap the entire field bandage. Wrap snugly, but do not pull excessively tight.

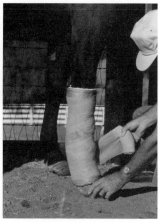

7A—Wrap the entire length of the field bandage. Use both rolls of gauze if desired.

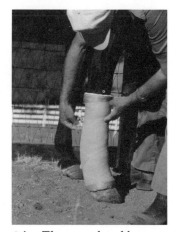

8A—The completed bandage. Secure the gauze wrapping with safety pins or with tape.

The second is the Robert-Jones bandage. The part of the horse most frequently in need of bandaging is the leg, below the hock or knee. There are many ways of doing this satisfactorily but, because I have seen so many legs damaged by improper bandaging (including some seriously bowed tendons), I am going to show what I consider to be the safest and most effective method—what is known as a Robert-Jones bandage. Due to the extremely thick layer of cotton padding used, there is very little danger of causing injury to the structures of the leg. At the same time, the compression caused by this bandage prevents edema and swelling in the limb. In addition, if there is drainage from a wound, the fluids are absorbed into the thick layer of cotton.

I use this bandage after suturing leg wounds, and leave it on for two weeks, until the sutures are ready to remove. It is also an excellent leg bandage for non-sutured wounds, preventing edema of the leg, supporting the limb, and absorbing discharge. I have even used it as a splint for certain fractures.

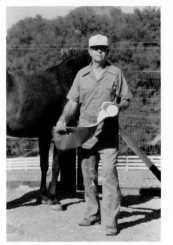

1R—First, unroll a full roll of absorbent cotton, removing the paper, and rerolling it without the paper.

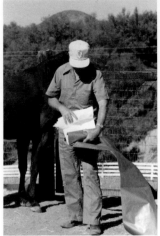

2R—Rerolling the cotton.

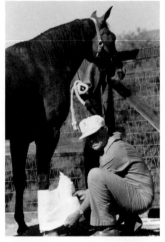

3R—Now you are ready to roll the cotton onto the leg. But first, cover any wounds with sterile gauze bandage, wrapping gently to avoid getting it too tight.

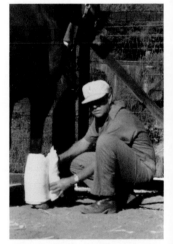

4R—Roll the entire roll of cotton around the leg from coronet to knee. It makes a big fat wad of cotton.

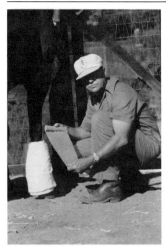

5R—Next, get a roll of four-inch roller gauze.

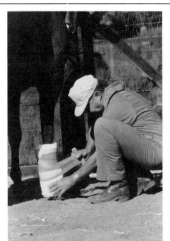

6R—And wrap it around the cotton from top to bottom. Pull it quite snug, but don't use excessive force or you will tear the gauze. As tight as possible without tearing the gauze is just right. Be sure not to go above or below the cotton. There should be an inch or so of cotton showing, top and bottom.

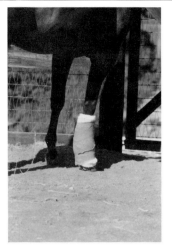

7R—Completed gauze wrap.

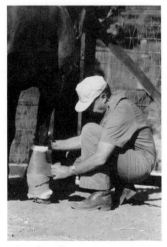

8R—Finally, using a strong elastic bandage (I am using Vetrap, but you can also use an Ace elastic bandage, or elastic adhesive bandage), wrap everything quite tightly. The cotton protects the circulation.

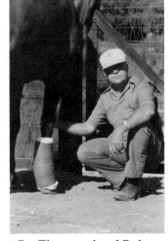

9R—The completed Robert-Jones bandage. When thumped with the finger it should sound like a ripe watermelon. Again, be sure there is a border of cotton padding at the top and bottom to prevent the outer bandage layer from cutting off circulation.

BANDAGING THE KNEE

It is often necessary to bandage a knee to cover a wound, or to hold a poultice in place. If the knee bandage is too loose, it will quickly fall down, or it will fail to hold the underlying dressing (which is covering the wound or the poultice) in place. If the knee bandage is too tight, it will cause pressure sores, especially at the back of the knee over the protruding accessory carpal bone. If a too-tight bandage compresses the upper portion of the flexor tendon, in back of and below the knee, it can bow the tendon.

The illustrated technique for bandaging the knee avoids these complications, and has served me well for many years.

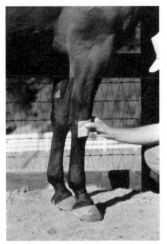

1K—First apply a dressing to the wound. In this case, we'll pretend that we have a puncture wound of the front of the knee that has been cleaned and disinfected. We cover the wound with an adaptic dressing.

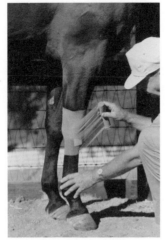

2K—Then a sterile four-inch cling gauze bandage is wrapped around the knee to cover the dressing. The gauze must be applied smoothly, with no wrinkles and snug enough to conform closely to the knee, but not too tight.

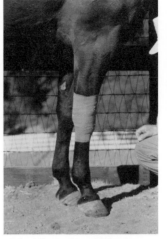

3K—The gauze roller bandage completely applied.

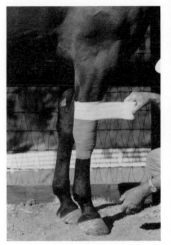

4K—Next, use elastic adhesive bandage and put a couple of wraps around the upper margin of the bandage, snugly, but not too tightly. The lower half of the tape sticks to the bandage, and the upper half to the hair on the forearm. This is what keeps the bandage from sliding down.

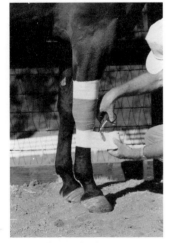

5K—Then, the lower margin of the bandage is similarly secured to the cannon. It is done exactly as the preceding step. This keeps the bandage from sliding upward.

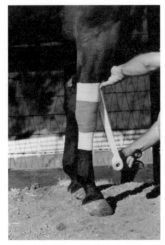

6K—A strip of elastic adhesive bandage is now run vertically, at the front of the knee.

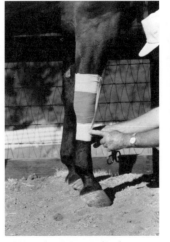

6K2—As it is applied, stretch it fully so that it will compress the bandage against the front of the knee. This important step will prevent gaping of the bandage as the knee flexes when the horse walks.

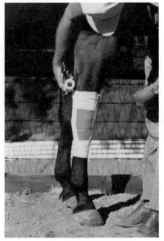

7K—Another vertical strip is placed at the back of the knee, as in the preceding step.

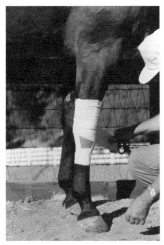

8K—A single layer of elastic adhesive bandage is now placed over everything, snugly, but not too tight.

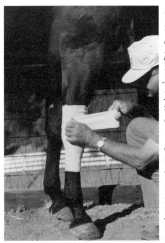

9K—This next step must be understood. Short strips of elastic bandage are now placed horizontally across the front of the underlying bandage. The strips extend from the middle of the outside of the leg to the middle of the inside of the leg. They do not go completely around the leg. Pull them as tightly as possible. They will cause compression at the front of the leg, but none behind the leg. Therefore, they do not cut off circulation. If you do not understand this step, omit it. It works beautifully if done correctly, but is dangerous if you do not understand it and wrap tightly completely around the leg.

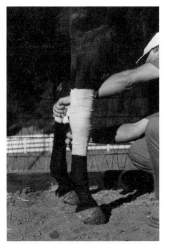

10K—Cutting the short strip should be done at the inside of the knee. I have pulled this short strip quite tight, and will run these short compressing strips along the entire front half of my bandage, from top to bottom.

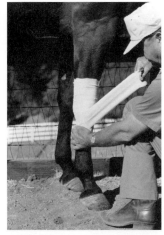

11K—Now wrap another layer of the elastic adhesive bandage over everything. Snug but not too tight.

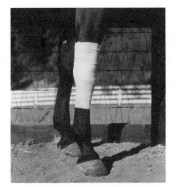

12K—The finished bandage. If done properly, it will not ride up or fall down, will not cut circulation, and will protect the dressing and injury beneath it, even if left on for one or two weeks.

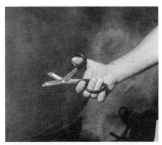

13K—To remove the bandage, you need a good sharp bandage scissors. These stainless steel German scissors with a plastic handle are excellent, and most veterinarians use them. Beware, however, of similar-looking but cheap imitations. The good ones are made in Germany.

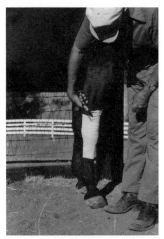

14K—Starting at the top, slide the lower blade of the scissors under the tape and cut downward.

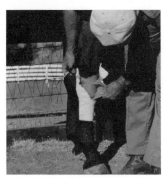

15K—Don't try to cut through all of the layers. They are too thick. Just concentrate on the tape, and perhaps one or two layers of gauze.

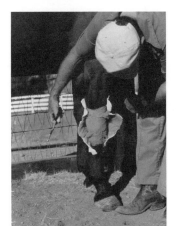

16K—The tape has been completely cut through.

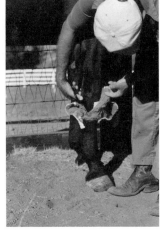

17K—Now finish cutting through the layers of gauze. The entire bandage is easily removed because it is only adherent to the hair of the horse at its top and bottom, along a two-inch-wide strip.

BANDAGING THE HOCK

Before reading this, read "Bandaging The Knee," because the same principles are involved, and they are more fully explained in the knee discussion.

The hock is very difficult to bandage because of its irregular shape and because it flexes so much when the horse moves. There are various techniques for bandaging the hock, but this method has worked well for me.

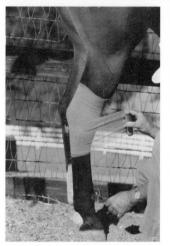

1H—We'll assume that the bandage is being applied to cover a wound, protected by a primary dressing such as gauze sponges, or an adaptic dressing. First, using four-inch cling gauze roller bandage, wrap the entire hock. Apply the gauze smoothly, without wrinkles, making it snug so as to conform to the hock, but not too tight. When completed it should look like the picture.

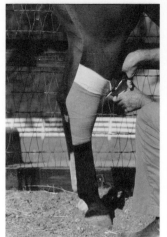

2H—Next, use elastic adhesive bandage to go around the leg, at the top of the bandage. The elastic adhesive bandage should stick to both the bandage and the hair of the leg. Use two or three layers. If the bandage is to stay on for a while, go higher up the leg to grab more hair. Snug, but not too tight.

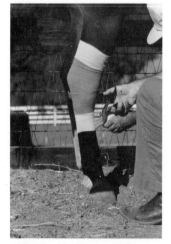

3H—Do the same at the lower edge of the gauze bandage.

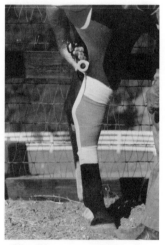

4H—Then run a vertical strip of elastic adhesive bandage at the back, covering the point of the hock. In large horses, use two or three overlapping strips. Stretch them tight when applying them. They will compress the back of the hock, prevent gaping of the bandage, and swelling of the point of the hock.

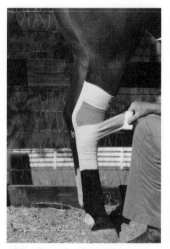

5H—Snugly, but not tightly, cover everything with a layer or two of the elastic adhesive tape. Expect to use two to three rolls when doing a hock.

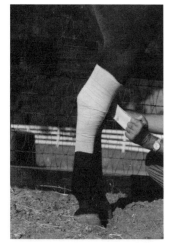

6H—Now, just as we did in bandaging the knee, we are going to very tightly apply short strips of tape halfway around the limb, but not all the way around. *Whether you place them at the front or back of the hock depends on where you want the pressure. If you are bandaging a wound or a lesion at the front of the hock, then put the pressure up front as I am doing here.*

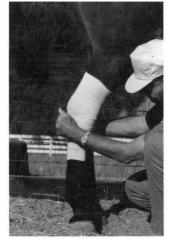

7H—But if you need the pressure behind the hock, then apply the short strips from the rear.

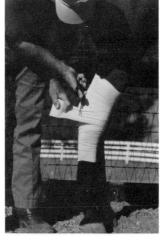

8H—Since you are only going halfway around the leg, you can stretch the elastic tape to its limit when you apply it, with no danger of cutting off the circulation to the lower leg. Lastly, cover all with a final layer of tape; not too tight.

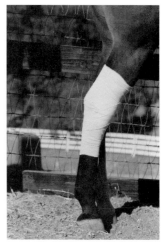

9H—The finished bandage. If done correctly, it will stay in place indefinitely. It conforms to the hock and applies pressure where needed without cutting off the circulation. Swelling of the limb below the bandage may mean that your bandage is too tight. If so, remove it and apply a new one.

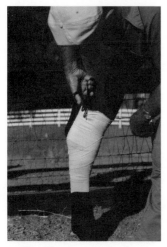

10H—To remove the bandage, see the instructions for the knee. Cut through the tape.

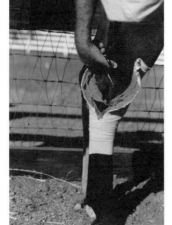

11H—Then cut through the gauze.

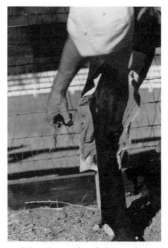

12H—Once both have been cut, peel the bandage off.

3 LAMENESS

For every instance of lameness, there is a cause. For some lamenesses, there are cures. For others, there are means of prevention.

Why It Happens

Why do horses have so much leg trouble? Why is lameness a leading problem to horse owners, and the treatment of lameness such an important part of veterinary practice? The answer is really a simple one. *Strain* causes most of the trouble. Just as an overloaded bridge collapses, or an overworked machine breaks down, so do the structures of the body give way when the load they are required to support overtaxes their capacity.

What are the causes of strain? They can be broken down into two general causes:

1/ Too much work for the part.
2/ Too little part for the work.

Let's consider the first cause: One of the qualities that has made the horse so valuable to man is his willingness to work. The horse doesn't quit when he is tired. He does not say, "I've had it. I can't do any more." Instead he keeps on going until he drops. It is, therefore, the rider's responsibility to protect the horse from overwork.

What kind of overwork is most common? Well, the leading mistake, in my opinion, is starting a horse too young. Riding a horse younger than three years of age is asking for trouble. I strongly insist that a colt should *not* be broken to ride until he is three years of age. In special cases you may give or take six months. For example, an extremely powerful and large Quarter Horse might be started at 30 months. Such horses mature early. On the other hand, a little

Photo by Pam Shewan

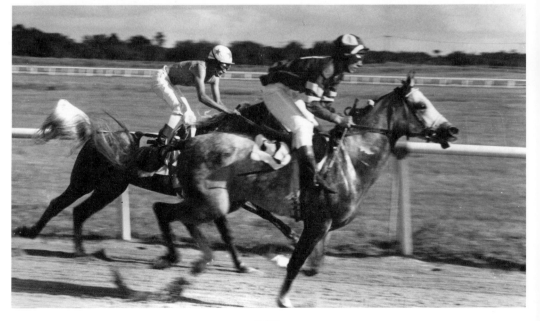

102

Arabian might be too young to start even after three years. Arabians mature slowly. Starting a horse too young is like putting an adolescent boy into a professional football training schedule. The bones, tendons, and ligaments are still soft and growing. They cannot take the gaff. Neither can the colt's. Strained young joints become inflamed. Ligaments rip the *periosteum* away from the underlying bone. Tendon fibers tear. Joint capsules stretch and swell. Later in life these injuries will scar and calcify. They will become chronically painful. In a cow or a dog or even a man, such injuries are uncomfortable but not serious. But in a horse they are vital injuries. A limping horse is useless as a riding animal. So stay off that colt until he grows up.

The one year of riding you gain by starting him at two may cost dearly later on. There is plenty of training you can give the colt between two and three without riding him. Work him from the ground. Teach him to back. Drive him with a pair of lines and teach him to turn. Teach him to ground tie, to be gentle. Handle his feet, his mouth, his ears. Teach him not to be afraid of a rope under his tail or between his legs. Teach him to load in a trailer and not to be afraid of fluttering objects and loud noises, and how to handle barbed wire. If you do not know how to train a colt, it will pay you to hire someone who does. Properly gentling a colt may save your front teeth later on and possibly your life. Waiting until he is three before riding him will save his legs.

When the colt is three, you may begin to ride him—but take it easy for that first year. For a full year, concentrate on basic things: stopping, reining, backing, handling his leads, etc. Not until he is four should hard work begin. Only now is his body beginning to toughen enough to stand a lifetime of constant strain. Not until the horse is four should he start his life's work, whether it be jumping, cutting, roping, stock horse and reining classes, barrel racing, gymkhana, and so on. I deplore the modern trend to jump on a two-year-old colt's back and immediately start teaching him to rope, cut cattle, or jump. It is two years too early. Such haste will be regretted a few years later. If horses were trained as I have outlined, we would see many more still actively competing past 20 years of age, and far fewer crippled at seven or ten years.

Now that I have covered the first cause—too much work for the part, let us regard the second—too little part for the work. By this, I am not especially discussing size. I am thinking of conformation. A small horse that is well built will hold up better than a big horse with such faults as crooked feet, sickled hocks, or pasterns that are either too long and sloping or excessively short and upright. Such weaknesses will break down under strain. Too many horses are evaluated by their color, head shape, and even their natural ability, while the vital structure of their legs is disregarded. What good is a "running heart" or "cow sense" in a horse with a set of ringbones, or a spavin the size of a turkey egg?

Another cause of "too little part for the work" is poor physical condition. Again we are not referring to quantity but quality. Everybody knows that it is foolhardy and dangerous for a person who has done no exercise for a year to go out and climb a mountain or run a quarter-mile race. Yet, we constantly see horses confined to a stall or corral for weeks, then taken out and ridden hard. Is it any wonder veterinarians are kept busy trying to repair the results of such foolishness. A horse must be physically conditioned to stand hard work without injury. He must be in shape. Being in good shape includes regular exercise, a correct diet, freedom from worms, and feet that are correctly trimmed and shod. Improper feeding, especially in colts, may result in skeletal weakness.

To summarize, select a horse with ideal conformation for the type of work he is going to do. If you must sacrifice conformation, do so elsewhere on his body, never on his limbs. Don't get on his back until he is a three-year-old. Don't work him hard until he is four. Keep him in hard physical condition, feed him correctly, shoe him properly. Respect his fatigue! If he does suffer a laming injury, have him examined by a competent veterinarian, and then follow the veterinarian's advice. Do these things and your horse will remain free of most common lamenesses.

Diagnosing

The most common diagnostic problem presented to the equine practitioner is lameness. In a general horse practice, the veterinarian may have to examine several lame horses every day. Therefore it should be of interest and value to the horse owner to understand how the veterinarian proceeds to diagnose the cause of lameness in a patient who cannot speak and tell "where it hurts."

When a lame horse is presented to us, usually the first thing we do is simultaneously ask for the history of the case while we look the patient over. The history must include several pertinent points:

1/ When did you first notice the lameness?

2/ Is it getting better, worse, or staying the same?

3/ Has he ever been lame before?

4/ What kind of work does he do?

5/ How old is he?

6/ How long have you owned him?

7/ What did he do before you owned him? Was he raced?

8/ Did the lameness come on gradually, or did it occur suddenly? Did he go lame during or after the last time he was ridden? How long afterward?

While the owner answers these questions, we'll walk around the horse to note his conformation. Is he well put together? Is he an athletic-looking individual? Is he delicate? Do his legs show evidence of much abuse? Are there weaknesses that would predispose lameness, such as being pigeon-toed or splay-footed; or having weak knees or weak tendons; or having pasterns that are too long, too short, too upright, or too angled?

Is he cow-hocked, straight-shouldered, sickle-hocked, curby, bow-legged, straight-stifled, or poorly muscled? Are his feet well shaped to absorb concussion? Are they too big, too small, too flat, or scarred from old injuries? Do the hoofs show concavity, or rings suggesting former laminitis?

Most important, are the feet atrophied or contracted, suggesting that the horse has been chronically favoring his feet? We are especially alerted if we see *one* foot more contracted than its mate. This is a common finding in chronic lameness. Often, long before the owner can detect lameness, the involved foot will start to shrink because it is getting less work than its mate.

After obtaining a history, and noting all of the above features as we briefly walk around the horse, we want to see the horse move out. Personally, I like to do this on a hard surface such as a paved blacktop road or driveway. I watch the horse walk a little ways, and then ask for a slow trot. Lameness is more obvious at a trot on a hard surface than under any other conditions. If there is a rider on the horse, it will also frequently accentuate the lameness, but the rider should keep a loose rein, sit easily, and preferably not post.

While the horse is trotted, we try to determine several things:

1/ Which leg is lame? Remember that the head goes *down* on the sound fore-leg, not on the lame one. The hip goes *down* on the good hind leg, not on the lame hind leg.

2/ Are the *other* legs sound? Frequently there is lameness in more than one leg, but the novice observer will only notice the one most severely lame.

3/ Does the horse move normally, aside from the limp? Is he coordinated? Does he flex and extend each joint freely? Does he take a full stride? Does he land flat-footed, or is he favoring the toe, or the heel? Does he stub his toes? Does circling in either direction accentuate the lameness?

Now, at last, we are ready to examine the horse more closely. We feel the affected leg. Is there fever anywhere? Can we palpate (feel) any swellings, or any painful spots? We apply pressure with the fingers; does he flinch when we press over the lateral cartilages? Are they flexible? Is there pain along the coronet?

Are the heels sore, or the suspensory ligaments? Does it hurt when we flex the ankle or the knee, or extend the elbow, or shoulder?

After cleaning the bottom of the foot, we check to see if there are any nails imbedded there. Is there any thrush? Are the grooves along the frog normal? Is the frog full and well formed?

We check the digital pulse; is it normal or increased and pounding? Perhaps that indicates inflammation within the foot.

Next, using special pincers called hoof

testers, or using a special hammer, we percuss and apply pressure to the various parts of the foot encased within the hoof wall, as well as the sole and frog. Does he flinch? Is that due to pain, or is he just nervous? Compare it with the sound foot to find out.

Sometimes even after all of the above procedures have been done, we are still unable to localize the cause of the lameness. If so, we resort to diagnostic blocking. Here, we block—with injections of a local anesthetic such as Novocain—the nerves to the various parts of the foot, just as the dentist deadens your teeth with a similar anesthetic.

We deaden the lowest nerve first. Then we test to be sure that part of the foot is numb. If it is, we trot the horse out. Is he still lame? If so, we block the next nerve . . . and the next one until, finally, the limp disappears. Now we know *where* the pain is.

Next, we must determine *what* is causing the pain in that location. This often necessitates X-ray studies. Acute bone injuries such as fractures can be readily detected with X-rays. Chronic bone injuries tend to build up calcium deposits. These, too, can be seen with X-rays. Fresh bone injuries other than fractures, such as bone bruises, are more difficult to detect.

Soft tissue injuries, such as sprains and strains, will show no X-ray changes while they are fresh, except for swelling. Later, when such injuries become chronic, they frequently develop visible calcium deposits.

Finally, after the diagnosis has been made and confirmed, specific treatment can be started.

Nerve Blocks

There are eleven veterinarians in my group practice. Four of us spend most of our time working with horses, but we treat all species of animals. It isn't unusual for one of our equine practitioners to be called in to offer a diagnostic opinion as to the cause of a lameness in a dog, cat, calf, or in some other species. This is because equine practitioners become particularly astute at diagnosing the cause of lameness. It is an important part of a horse practice.

In diagnosing lameness and its cause,

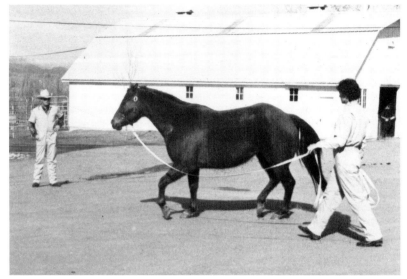

A flat, hard surface aids in diagnosing lameness.

the veterinarian first tries to get an accurate history of the lameness, paying attention to its duration, its pattern, its intensity, and any factors that the client thinks are pertinent. The veterinarian will then ask questions that will provide further information.

Next, the doctor will watch the horse move. Depending on the severity of the lameness, he or she may want the horse to be moved about in various ways, on various surfaces or inclines, and at varying gaits. This can be done in hand, at liberty on a longe line, or under saddle or in harness.

The conformation of the horse is observed. There might be significant conformational defects that can lead to lameness; or there might be atrophy or wasting of a foot or upper limb that indicates a long-standing lameness. Often, visible swelling or enlargement of a part offers an important diagnostic clue.

Finally, the veterinarian will feel the leg, pick it up, and check for swelling, heat, pain, or a loss of range of motion. The lame leg might be compared to the opposite leg in order to evaluate that particular horse's individual reactions. The joints are flexed, and pressure is placed on the anatomic structures with the fingers and the hands, and with instruments like a hoof tester.

By this time, the veterinarian can usually make a diagnosis, or is at least able to localize the problem to a specific area (foot, ankle, knee, etc.), and narrow the diagnosis to a few possibilities.

Often, more than one problem is identified, and it becomes a question of *which* of the problems is causing the actual lameness. Sometimes two or even three problems exist in a single limb.

Frequently the client tells us that the lameness appeared recently, but that's because he or she didn't notice it until recently. In reality, our examination clearly indicates a long-standing chronic problem. We can determine this by irregular shoe wear, and the presence of atrophy (shrinkage or wasting) in the hoof, or in the muscles of the upper limb.

At this point, the cause may be obvious enough for the vet to make a positive diagnosis and start treatment. In other cases, the area of pain may be obvious to the diagnostician, but X-ray studies will be necessary to rule out bone damage, to determine the extent of the lesion, or to find out which specific structures are involved.

In many cases, however, the veterinarian is stumped before he reaches this point. He might know *where* the pain is, but he might not know exactly which part is involved. For example, he might know the problem is in the hoof, but is not able to tell whether the toe or heel is involved.

Sometimes, as I said earlier, the vet finds several problem areas; however, he can't tell which of the problem areas is actually causing the limp because he is dealing with a patient who cannot talk. And, sometimes, especially with a stoic patient, the examiner simply cannot get the horse to show a pain reaction no matter where he pokes and probes. At the other extreme, there is the fearful, hypersensitive horse who acts like *everything* hurts when he is examined.

For patients like these, the veterinarian will utilize diagnostic nerve blocking. Using a local anesthetic such as Novocaine, Lidocaine, or Carbocaine, the vet will block out the nerves to various parts of the hoof or limb. After each block, the horse will be re-examined for lameness. When the limp suddenly disappears or dramatically lessens, the vet knows *where* the lameness is located. The next step, then, is usually X-raying to determine what is going on.

Since our patients can't talk (although their behavior and appearance tell us a lot), diagnostic nerve blocking is an extremely important technique for the equine practitioner. Obviously, it requires an expert knowledge of anatomy to do nerve blocking, and experience to properly interpret its results.

Nerve blocking, however, is not 100 percent effective. But then, nothing in medical practice ever is. For nerve blocking to be significant, the patient must, first of all, be obviously lame. If the lameness is vague, or if it is intermittent, the results of a block cannot be considered significant.

Secondly, a reliable block must be obtained. This means that the proper amount of the anesthetic solution must be placed in or close to the nerve. The results of the block must be tested. If the area is not *desensitized* after the block, then it cannot be expected to arrest the lameness. Many of us have had the experience of having the dentist block the nerve to a tooth, only to find that there is still feeling in the tooth when he starts drilling.

It must be realized that time is a factor. It sometimes takes five or ten minutes, or even longer, for a block to take full effect. Too, the block will start to wear off after a while, somewhere between 20 minutes and an hour.

Lastly, nerve patterns vary. We are not all "constructed" by the book. There are often nerve branches supplying a part that are missed during a routine block, necessitating re-blocking at a higher level. So, a lot of skill and experience are involved, not only in *doing* the nerve block, but in *interpreting* it.

Most experienced horse owners are familiar with diagnostic nerve blocking, and I hope this article will help them, as well as inexperienced horse owners, to understand the procedure.

Here are two case histories from our clinic in which nerve blocking played a role. They show how helpful this procedure can be.

Case No. 1

History: A seven-year-old gelding, intermittently lame in left fore.
Exam: Seems to go short on both forelegs, but more obviously in left. Slight atrophy left fore heel. Vague discomfort when pressure is applied to both fore frogs.
Nerve blocking: The left fore posterior digital lateral (outside heel) nerve is blocked. There is a 50 percent improvement in the lameness.

The left fore posterior digital medial (inside heel) nerve is blocked. The horse now goes 100 percent sound on the left fore, and after 15 minutes, the right fore appears lame.
Tentative diagnosis: Navicular disease of both forefeet, more severe in the left. Confirmed by radiography (X-ray).

Case No. 2

History: A ten-year-old mare; low-grade chronic lameness in the right fore.
Exam: Slight loss of range of motion when ankle is flexed. Obvious sidebones. Old knee injury with enlargement and slight loss of range of motion. Moderate atrophy of the foot. Several problem areas can be seen.
Radiography: Reveals well-developed sidebones, early ringbone in the pastern joint, and a little calcium formation in the knee. The question: Which of these problems is causing the lameness?
Nerve blocking: No improvement in lameness after both heel nerves are blocked. This rules out the sidebones as the cause of the lameness. After the outside nerve just above the fetlock is blocked, there is partial improvement. When the entire limb, from the fetlock down, is blocked, there is 100 percent improvement.
Diagnosis: It looks like the ringbone is causing the problems. The old knee injury is obviously not a factor.

Splints

Millions of years ago, the earliest known ancestor of the horse roamed the earth. He was the size of a small dog, and had five toes on each foot. His descendants gave rise to many varieties of hoofed mammals we know today. Among these were the first primitive horses. These were small, three-toed creatures.

As countless centuries passed, two of the toes, along with their associated bones, receded, and the horse became a one-toed animal. The single toe, covered with a tough hoof, was better suited for travel over the arid plains that are the horse's natural environment. The two toes that disappeared left vestiges that are still part of the modern horse's anatomy. The ergot is a vestigial toe, and will be found in the tuft of hair at the back of the fetlock. The chestnut is a vestigial toe, and is that piece of hoof material found on the inner surface of the horse's upper leg.

If you will look at the leg of a horse skeleton, you will notice the evolutionary results of what were once five metacarpal or metatarsal bones. (In humans these five bones may be felt in the hand or foot, respectively.) In the horse, the first and fifth (outermost and innermost) metacarpals have completely disappeared. The middle metacarpal has grown thick and strong and forms what we call the cannon bone. We should point out that in the forelegs, we speak of the metacarpal region, and in the hind legs we call it the metatarsal region. For simplification in this article we will just speak of metacarpal bones.

What about the second and fourth metacarpal bones? What happened to them? Well, they may still be found, shortened, thinned, non-functional, but very much in evidence. They lie on either side of the cannon bone, toward the back, and are closely attached to that important main leg bone. These two bones are known as the splint bones.

In young horses, the splint bones are rather loosely attached to the cannon bone. By five or six years of age, this attachment has usually calcified, and the bones are firmly fused. In young horses, the attachments sometimes become inflamed and painful. If this inflammation is allowed to go unchecked, the body responds by excessive calcification. The inflamed area gradually develops into a hard, bony mass. This mass appears as an unsightly hard lump on the cannon bone, and horsemen for centuries have termed it a splint.

Since splints are caused by inflammation of the attachment between the splint bones, it is important to study the causes of such inflammation. The most common cause is movement between the bones during strenuous exercise. In other words, work may strain a young horse, whereas the same effort in a mature horse with fully developed bones may do no harm. Such splint strains may be caused by fast turns and stops, concussion by hard road surfaces or jumping, and crooked feet due to poor conformation or poor shoeing. Splint injuries are also caused by a blow, such as from an opposite foot. Lastly, some very young horses develop splints due to nutritional bone disease. Nutritional bone disease is seen in young horses fed inadequate diets, vitamin-deficient diets, or excessive vitamin and mineral supplementation.

Any portion of any splint bone may develop a splint. Remember that each leg has two splint bones, making a total of eight per horse. However, the great majority of splints occur on the inside of the front legs. Some are up high, close to the knee. Others occur lower down, some in the lower third of the cannon.

Since most splints are due to strain, it is understandable that the heavy breeds are more predisposed than lighter horses.

Splints don't often cause lameness except in the early stages. At this point, no swelling may be visible, but the area involved will be tender if pressed. Lameness is more severe after a workout. In time the splint calcifies and the hard bump develops. With this, lameness usually disappears, and thereafter, the splint is considered a blemish rather than an unsoundness.

An exception is the "pegged splint." This is a splint that goes around the back of the leg impinging on the suspensory ligament, flexor tendon, or carpal joint, thereby causing permanent lameness. But pegged splints are rare.

Most splints, once healed, are not as important a defect as many horsemen consider them to be. Their greatest significance is that they indicate strain or malnutrition early in life. It is possible for an old "cold," painless splint to flare up if rapped or otherwise reinjured.

Splints are, as you can see, not too difficult to diagnose, except perhaps when first developing. We do like to X-ray them, however, in order to differentiate simple splints from a fracture of the splint bone. A fractured splint can be a stubborn problem, and some of the treatments used for ordinary splints will worsen a fracture.

Old, chronic splints are best left alone, unless pegged. The only chance of removing a pegged splint is to remove it surgically.

Early splints should be treated, because by stopping them, it is often possible to prevent the disfiguring enlargement that lessens the value of the horse.

Veterinarians use several techniques to control early splints. One method is to cauterize the splint deeply, right to the bone. Another method is periosteotomy, which involves incising the membrane covering the splint bone. Diathermy has been used on some cases. Another method is to subdue the inflammation by injecting cortisone under the periosteum (bone membrane cover) at the splint site.

Regardless of the method used, the horse should be rested, and put on a balanced ration. Pasture rest is usually ideal. The feet should be kept trimmed.

Stumbling

We veterinarians often have horses presented to us with a complaint of stumbling. Such a horse stumbles frequently at any or all gaits; there is no apparent lameness; the horse may at times fall to his knees, or even go clear down with a rider; and the stumbling is most apparent under saddle, or when the horse is being led. In most cases, the horse does not stumble when loose or running free, but there are exceptions, as we shall see.

The owner is justifiably concerned when a horse stumbles repeatedly. Such a horse is no pleasure to ride, and can be extremely dangerous.

What causes such stumbling? In the absence of actual lameness, stumbling can be caused by a number of things.

Some horses stumble because they are inherently lazy. They don't pick up their feet, and therefore stub their toes over every irregularity in the ground. Usually such a horse stumbles mostly at a walk, less at a trot, and rarely at a lope (when he is alert). This kind of horse tends to carry his head low, with his nose out. It will help to collect this horse, to gather him up, to bit him up, to teach him flexion, and to get him to work off his hindquarters. Rolling the toe of the shoe may reduce his stumbling, but weighting the forefeet will increase his knee action more effectively.

Stumbling is also seen in some base-narrow horses. These horses are massive through the shoulders, broad of chest, and have front legs that taper inward towards the ground, often terminating in pigeon-toed feet. Such horses are often heavy on the forehand, and lack agility in front. They may sometimes be called "muscle-bound." They paddle out when they travel. Now, I realize that many good horses are built this way, and many of them never stumble and are superb athletes. Yet, certain stumblers do fit this description. I sometimes wonder if the stumbling factor involves the ratio between chest width and leg length. Personally, I like to see a long shoulder on a horse, and *depth* of chest rather than a lot of width through the front end.

One of the most common causes of stumbling is poor coordination. Some horses, like some people, simply lack coordination. They are awkward and graceless, and have poor control over their movements. There's no cure for this kind of horse, and there is one thing about this kind of horse I'd like to point out.

He may not necessarily *look* like a poor athlete. He may be well bred, and of pleasing conformation, and still be a bad stumbler. Again, we can use the human analogy. There are well-built people who are *not* good athletes, and there are people who are *not* well built who have excellent coordination, fast reflexes, a reasonable amount of strength, and who are quite good athletically. Ideally, of course, we like to see a horse that has both good conformation and good performance ability.

Some horses stumble because they have suffered damage to the central nervous system (brain or spinal cord). Neck and back injuries often produce "wobbler" horses. Such horses travel awkwardly and in an uncoordinated manner. The symptoms are usually manifested more in the hindquarters, but sometimes these horses will have difficulty up front, causing them to stumble and even cross their front legs when they move. Certain diseases, like sleeping sickness, and certain poisons, like loco weed, can also permanently damage the central nervous system.

Next, we must consider the horse that stumbles because of chronic foot pain. He may not show an obvious limp if both front feet, for example, hurt equally. Instead, he carries as much weight as possible on his hindquarters, and tends to stub his toes and stumble. The most common example of this kind

of unsoundness is navicular disease. The horse's heels hurt, so he travels "up" on his toes, stumping along and kicking up little puffs of dust with the toes of his forefeet. If the ground is irregular, stumbling will occur at the *end* of the stride.

Shoulder lameness will also cause a horse to stumble, because the shoulder pain makes it difficult for the horse to fully extend his arm. Such a horse has a very short stride, and he will stumble at the *beginning* of the stride.

A horse may also stumble due to weakness resulting from fatigue, illness, anemia, or heart disease.

Finally, stumbling can be temporarily caused by poor shoeing. If the feet are unbalanced, trimmed at an improper angle, or are carrying shoes of improper weight or poor fit, stumbling can result. In fact, corrective shoeing is the most important thing we can do for the stumbling horse after he has been examined, the cause of stumbling determined, and the cause removed if possible. If the stumbling cannot be totally eliminated, the horse must be regarded as unsound and unsafe to ride.

Laminitis and Founder

Nearly every horseman is familiar with the term *founder*, but do you really understand what the term means? I will try to explain as simply as possible what founder is and what can be done about it, but before I do, I must impress three very important points on you.

1/ Founder (also called laminitis) can be prevented. A foundered horse is always the result of some person's carelessness or lack of knowledge.

2/ A neglected case of founder ruins a horse for life. It is incurable!

3/ Founder is a common disease. Veterinarians engaged in an equine practice see many foundered horses. So don't think that it cannot happen to your horse.

Now, to explain the basic disorders that occur in this very complex disease, when a horse founders, many changes take place in his body, but, most important, there is a great pressure, and congestion of blood in certain blood vessels. There is a fever, the horse sweats and breathes rapidly, and the membranes of the eyes and nose are flushed and hot.

If the stumbling cannot be totally eliminated, the horse must be regarded as unsound and unsafe to ride.

Elsewhere in the body the congested blood vessels do not result in serious damage as a rule, but in the feet, encased in a solid casing of hoof, the pressure causes excruciating pain (ever smash your thumbnail with a hammer?) and the *laminae*, the sensitive inner hoof tissues, are permanently damaged. Thus, after the acute laminitis subsides, the feet, in time, become increasingly deformed. The sole drops, the wall separates, the toe turns out, and we see the typical, ringed, abnormal feet of a horse with chronic founder.

Usually, in chronic founder, the coffin bone, having detached at least partially from the hoof wall, rotates downward. However, this is not always true. In some cases the entire coffin bone simply drops without rotating. We call these cases "sinkers," and they are a very serious form of founder requiring skillful corrective shoeing.

What are the causes of founder?

1/ Overloading on grain or lush grass.

2/ Drinking cold water when overheated, or otherwise causing rapid changes in body temperature—for example, bathing a hot horse with cold water, or standing a hot horse in a chilling wind. If you will think about it, you can see how such sudden chilling of large areas of the body can send excessive blood rushing to the extremities.

3/ Concussion during work on hard roads, especially paved roads.

4/ Exhaustion, especially when in an unconditioned animal.

5/ Untreated infections, such as pneumonia, and infection of the uterus (foaling founder or parturient laminitis).

6/ Acute allergic reactions (actually this includes most grain founders).

7/ Increased weight on the feet, as when one leg is lame, or shifting back and forth when traveling by sea. Naturally, the overweight animal founders more easily than the one in proper condition.

8/ Drastic laxatives.

9/ Heat stroke.

If you will read the above list again, you will see why proper management and intelligent horsemanship prevent founder.

A foundered horse requires prompt treatment. Drugs have been discovered that are of great value.

Only time will tell if the horse with laminitis can be saved by treatment or if the feet will suffer permanent damage.

Many horses with chronic founder are not too severely affected and can lead useful lives if correctly shod with special shoes.

Corrective shoeing can be the salvation of a foundered horse. There are a variety of founder shoes. Most of them are designed to correct rotation of the coffin bone and protect the dropped sole. Foundered feet sometimes need reconstructive surgery.

Currently, the heart-bar shoe and the adjustable heart-bar shoe are in vogue for foundered horses. If correctly made by a farrier trained in their use, they can offer dramatic relief to the foundered horse.

I might add that veterinarians see many, many horses with *mild* chronic founders and often the owner and even the blacksmith are not aware of the situation. Such horses commonly go sound except when barefoot. They then quickly go very lame as the hoof wall breaks away and weight is brought to bear on the abnormally flat sole.

Once again, we see a disease, both serious and common, that is *preventable* if we think and follow the rules.

Periostitis

The next time you have barbecued ribs, take a look at that thin layer of membrane that lies between the meat and the bone. This membrane is called the periosteum, which means, literally, around the bone. The periosteum protects and nourishes the bone, and serves as an anchor for ligaments and tendons. It is also involved in bone growth, especially in young animals, by virtue of a layer of special bone-forming cells. The last function is important, as we shall soon see.

Like any tissue in the body, the periosteum may be injured. When it is injured, inflammation sets in and then we say that a *periostitis* has occurred. The injury might be a blow, such as a kick in the shins. Or, it might be a strain. As an example of the latter, suppose a young horse is worked too hard. That bit of periosteum where a tendon or ligament is attached is overworked. It is injured.

It therefore becomes inflamed. A periostitis has set in. It is painful, therefore the horse limps. The blood supply increases and the part becomes swollen and feverish. This stimulates bone-forming cells that start to form excessive bone. What is the end result? A bony enlargement.

Many of the common leg lamenesses and unsoundnesses that you are familiar with are wholly, or mostly, a simple periostitis. You probably weren't aware that a periostitis was involved, because the common names do not indicate it. These common names originated long ago, and the horsemen who thought them up had no idea that all they were talking about was periostitis.

Now let's list some of the common periostitis lesions of the horse's leg:

Bucked shins: A periostitis at the front of the cannon bone. It occurs almost exclusively in the front legs of racing colts, soon after training begins, and is due to strain caused by excessive demand on immature legs. Bucked shins appear as a warm swelling at the front of the cannon bone, accompanied by pain and lameness.

Osselets: Periostitis at the front of the fetlock. Osselets are most common in young race horses for the same reasons cited above. Neglected or persistent cases may eventually involve the underlying bone and cause arthritis (inflammation of a joint) of the fetlock with resulting calcification, stiffness, and chronic pain.

Ringbone: This term is applied to several abnormalities of the pastern region. There may be periostitis alone, or periostitis plus arthritis. Ringbone is very common in all kinds of horses and can appear at any age. X-ray studies are valuable in determining the kind of ringbone present, the amount of damage present, the chances for cure, and the best method of treatment. Advanced cases with abundant bony enlargement encircling the pastern gave rise to the common name of ringbone, but it is important to understand that early cases, and even some advanced cases, do not show the "ring" of bone. Sometimes the owner is surprised by the veterinarian's diagnosis of ringbone when no ring can be seen.

Splints: These begin as a simple periostitis of the splint bones. Later, new bone growth (exostosis) results from stimulation of the periosteum, and the result is a hard, unsightly, bony enlargement.

Pyramidal disease: Also known as *buttress foot* or *extensor process disease.* It begins as a periostitis of the foot, causing enlargement in the area of the coronet (top of the hoof). It is often confused with low ringbone. As in most cases of advanced periostitis, new bone growth appears that causes deformity. Also, as is true of most periostitis allowed to progress unimpeded, the underlying bone becomes involved (osteitis) and thereby weakened. In pyramidal disease, the new bone, or the weakened extensor process, may fracture, worsening the lameness.

The above are just a few of the more common examples of periostitis in the horse. Now let's emphasize some of the important aspects of periostitis, keeping in mind what we have learned about the tissue involved (periosteum) and the changes that occur in that tissue when it is inflamed.

1/ Periostitis can occur any time the periosteum is injured. The injury can be a blow, strain due to overwork, or weakness of the part caused by poor conformation or malnutrition.

2/ Periostitis is painful. In the limbs, therefore, it can cause lameness. Since periosteum contains bone-forming cells, periostitis can cause the growth of unwanted new bone. Such bony enlargements are often impossible to remove. Therefore, it is important to diagnose periostitis as early as possible so that prompt treatment can stop the inflammation before permanent damage is done. Early diagnosis depends on skilled examination, and the value of X-ray studies is obvious, because they often reveal the presence of periostitis long before it is obvious to the examiner's eye or hand.

3/ *Early* periostitis—before new bone has formed—is an inflammation, characterized by heat, pain, and swelling. Accordingly, the treatment of *early* periostitis is anti-inflammatory. We therefore employ rest, cold, astringents, and anti-inflammatory drugs at this stage, when the fire is burning bright.

4/ *Chronic* periostitis, with calcification and new bone growth requires dif-

Understand that the limbs of the horse, like your own, are composed of bones, joints, muscles, tendons, ligaments, bursas, blood vessels, nerves, and skin.

ferent treatment. The smoldering inflammation must be stopped if possible, and an attempt is made to promote the absorption of new bone. This is difficult and often impossible to achieve. Towards that end, such treatments are used as counter-irritation with stimulant blistering agents or cautery, X-ray therapy, or ultrasound.

5/ *Advanced* periostitis may involve underlying bone or adjacent structures. Thus, the underlying bone may become involved, causing osteitis. Or, an adjacent joint may become involved, causing arthritis. These changes further complicate an already serious process.

6/ Try to think intelligently and scientifically of all lamenesses in the horse. Understand that the limbs of the horse, like your own, are composed of bones, joints, muscles, tendons, ligaments, bursas, blood vessels, nerves, and skin. I use technical terms, such as periostitis, arthritis, bursitis, and tendonitis, not because they sound impressive, but because they tell us exactly which structure is diseased. This, therefore, helps us to intelligently understand what is wrong and how to correct it. The old horseman's terms of bowed tendon, popped knee, ringbone, curb, and osselet, etc., are traditional and convenient, but, unfortunately, they don't explain what exactly is wrong and, therefore, encourage improper or harmful treatment.

Sidebones

Feel the foot of a young, healthy horse. On either side of the foot, back toward the heel and above the coronet, you can find a firm, moveable, resilient structure. These are the lateral cartilages. If these cartilages ossify, or calcify, and turn into bone, they are called sidebones.

Sidebones are often blamed for causing lameness in horses. It is true that a sidebone *can* cause lameness, but many horses have sidebones that do not cause any trouble at all. It is not unusual for the lateral cartilages to ossify into bone as a horse gets older. This is especially true in heavy, big-boned horses such as heavy hunters or those of draft breeding.

Concussion—pounding on hard surfaces—is believed to cause sidebones. Conformation faults can also contribute

to ossification of the lateral cartilages. For example, a horse that toes in or stands pigeon-toed is prone to develop sidebones on the outside of the foot. Conversely, a horse that toes out is more likely to develop sidebones on the inside of the foot. But outside sidebones are more common.

Heredity, too, seems to play a role in determining whether or not sidebones will develop, and it is possible that nutritional factors also exist.

Sidebones occur most often in the front feet, probably because they bear more of the horse's weight than do the hind feet.

Wire cuts often extend to and lacerate the lateral cartilage. After such an injury heals, it is not unusual for the cartilage to turn to bone.

Horses that have been foundered or have contracted heels due to poor shoeing, or have excessively straight pasterns are also predisposed to sidebones—probably because the hoof deformity that exists in these cases renders the foot less able to absorb concussion properly.

As we pointed out earlier, most sidebones do not cause much trouble, although they are sometimes blamed for lameness due to some other, less obvious cause. Even when sidebones *do* cause lameness, it is often a temporary problem.

A sidebone can join a ringbone, causing a serious lameness. Or, a sidebone, being brittle and less flexible than a normal lateral cartilage, can fracture. A fractured sidebone may heal with rest, but sometimes surgery is necessary.

When sidebones cause lameness, ordinary corrective shoeing may be very helpful. The quarters of the hoof wall are grooved or rasped thin to make the foot more flexible at the heel, thereby relieving some of the pressure over the sidebone. It may also help to roll the toe, and set the nails well forward. Of course, there are pain-relieving drugs that can be used, but these offer only temporary relief. When all else fails, a low neurectomy may allow the horse to continue working, at least for a while.

Ringbone

A horse is said to have ringbone when bony growths (extoses) develop in the pastern or coffin joint areas. Technically the actual lesions consist of a periostitis (inflammation of the membrane covering the bone with eventual outgrowth of new bone), or an osteoarthritis (inflammation of the joint, with eventual outgrowth of new bone)—or a combination of both conditions.

Ringbone is caused by injury. The most common type of injury is strain that damages the ligaments attached to the bone. Poor conformation contributes to such strains. For example, a horse that toes in or toes out, or a horse with short, upright pasterns, will suffer more ankle strain than will a "well-engineered" horse. Such horses are therefore more prone to develop ringbone. Ringbone is thought to be inheritable, but it is possible that all that is actually inherited are the conformation faults that predispose the horse to ringbone.

Ringbone can be caused by injuries other than strains. A deep wire cut often results in a ringbone. Blows that bruise the bone can also produce ringbone. Small fractures, particularly of the extensor process of the third phalanx, can lead to serious ringbone. Malnutrition early in life may later cause ringbone.

We often hear of high or low ringbone, or of true or false ringbone. A high ringbone is around or near the pastern joint. Such ringbones are sometimes huge, but if the joint itself is not involved, there may be little or no lameness associated with it.

Low ringbone is around or near the coffin joint. It is especially common at the front of the foot, involving the extensor process of the third phalanx. Because low ringbone occurs under the coronet, within the confines of the hoof, the pain and subsequent lameness it causes can be severe, even though the lesion is very small and not at all apparent when the foot is viewed. Of course, the lesion is visible on X-ray pictures. Chronic low ringbone involving the pyramidal process (extensor process of the third phalanx) is called pyramidal disease. The coronet begins to bulge in such a case, and such a foot is called a *buttress foot*.

Many horses have naturally knobby joints, and it is easy to confuse them with ringbone. X-ray studies clearly show the difference.

When lameness is caused by ringbone, the diagnosis is sometimes easy. There may be obvious heat, pain, and swelling over the ringbone. In other cases the symptoms are more subtle. The diagnostician watches for a characteristic gait, pain, or flexion, or digital pressure, and the response to diagnostic nerve blocks. X-ray studies are very useful, and absolutely essential to rule out fractures.

"True" ringbone involves the joints and is more painful than "false" ringbone, which involves only the bone between the joints. Such distinctions are a bit confusing because what is important is whether or not the horse is lame or going to be lame.

When ringbone can be diagnosed in the *very early* stages, when it is limited to a periostitis, and actual arthritis has not yet developed, it may heal with strict rest, which can be best enforced with a cast. This is often combined with the use of anti-inflammatory drugs.

I have had good results in treating early ringbone with deep cautery (firing), as recommended by Dr. O.R. Adams in his book, *Lameness in Horses.*

Low ringbone is always more serious than high ringbone. High chronic ringbone sometimes responds to surgical fusion of the joint.

Corrective shoeing of horses with true lameness-causing ringbone is rarely satisfactory in saddle horses. In the old days, the use of special shoes such as a full-roller-motion shoe might have allowed a draft horse to work by transforming a severe lameness to a slight lameness. But such partial improvement is inadequate in saddle horses. In my experience, corrective shoeing is most useful when a healed case of beginning ringbone is put back to work. Then, proper shoeing may help prevent a relapse.

The most common mistake I see in ringbone is neglect. Frequently a young, good horse develops a little lameness from a very early ringbone. If the case was immediately diagnosed, treated, and rested, a cure might be possible. Instead, the owner keeps the horse working and fools around with liniments and pain-relieving drugs, and soon the case has progressed to the point where it is incurable. It is so foolish to risk a horse's entire future in order to make another show, or win one more trophy.

Sweeny

Many puzzling and obscure lamenesses in horses are blamed on the shoulder. "I think it's his shoulder, Doc," is an opinion frequently offered to the veterinarian when he arrives to examine a horse for lameness. Usually, the problem turns out to be down in the foot. However, shoulder problems *do* occur in horses, and the most common one we see is the condition known as *sweeny*.

Sweeny refers to the atrophy, or shrinking, of the shoulder muscles. In fact, the term has been applied to atrophy of *any* muscle in the horse. For example, a horse with atrophy of the hip muscles may be said to have "sweeny of the hip." But generally, when horsemen speak of a sweeny, they refer to that shoulder lameness characterized by wasting of the muscles over the shoulder blade and shoulder joint.

Classically, the disease is caused by a blow to the point of the shoulder. The *suprascapular* nerve crosses the point of the shoulder, and if the nerve is injured, sweeny will result. The muscles over the shoulder blade, the *infraspinatus* and *supraspinatus* muscles, are supplied by this nerve. As the muscles atrophy, they greatly shrink in size, causing a hollow appearance to the shoulder. The spine of the shoulder blade sticks out prominently, instead of being concealed as it normally is by the muscle masses above and below it.

As a horse runs through a gate he may bump a shoulder to cause sweeny. Or he may run into a post or a tree. A kick by another horse can cause sweeny. In the old days, pressure from an ill-fitting collar caused sweeny in draft horses.

It is important to understand that atrophy of a muscle can be caused not only by nerve damage, but also by lack of use. Therefore, *any* lameness that causes the horse not to use his shoulder muscles may lead to sweeny. However, if the cause of the pain can be removed, and the horse encouraged to use the shoulder, the sweeny will reverse itself. Even where actual nerve damage exists, recovery is possible. Nerve tissue heals slowly, but it is capable of healing. In such cases, it is important to keep the muscle alive and healthy lest it be irreversibly atrophied while the nerve repairs itself.

As a rule, if a shoulder injury is followed by *complete* atrophy of the shoulder muscles in less than two weeks, there is usually said to be hopeless nerve damage. Perhaps in the future, operations on the nerve itself can save such horses from permanent sweeny. In cases where there is only partial atrophy of the muscles, there is more hope.

When a crushing blow to the point of the shoulder occurs, the treatment of most immediate value is the application of ice packs to the point of the shoulder. The use of anti-inflammatory drugs may be useful to prevent excessive swelling and destruction to the nerve. When severe sweeny develops, stimulation of the shoulder muscles may help to keep that structure vital while the nerve heals. This may involve passive exercises, massage, and the use of a galvanic electric stimulator to cause contraction of the muscle fibers, thereby exercising them.

Blistering, or firing the shoulder, has been a traditional form of treatment, but an ineffective one.

No case of sweeny should be considered as absolutely hopeless until half a year has gone by. Some cases will improve after one or two months.

Chronic cases of sweeny have been treated with injections of irritating chemicals that cause the shoulder muscles to swell; this may cause them to *look* more normal, but does not actually improve their disability.

Many sweenied horses can travel quite sound after they learn to compensate for their handicap.

I have had spectacular results in several severely sweenied horses after injecting the involved shoulder joint with long-acting cortisone-type drugs. These experiences have led me to believe that perhaps more cases of sweeny are due to severe pressure from within the shoulder joint, rather than bruising or contusion of the suprascapular nerve itself.

An example occurred when an Arabian stallion crashed into the judges' stand at a show, suffering a shoulder injury. Severe sweeny promptly followed, and the owners were very discouraged. I saw the horse about a week or so after the injury, and after taking X-ray pictures to rule out a fracture, I injected the joint. The lameness swiftly improved, and the sweeny completely disappeared.

Encouraged by the results in this case, I treated two more fresh sweeny cases, and again observed prompt recovery. I began to wonder if this treatment would be of value in a more chronic case. In 1970 a polo mare was involved in a collision with another horse during a match. The other horse was killed, and the mare suffered a sweenied left shoulder. I saw her two months after the accident. She was badly sweenied and so, after giving the owner little hope for recovery, I injected the shoulder. She was so greatly improved that three weeks later, I repeated the injection. The mare recovered completely and returned to full use.

Subsequently, I have treated numerous cases and most of them responded similarly.

I doubt if this kind of treatment would be of value in a sweeny more than, say, six months old. But certainly in any recent case, this type of treatment is worth trying.

Injection of the shoulder joint requires a long needle and an expert knowledge of anatomy. It should only be performed by a qualified veterinarian, using careful precautions to minimize the possibility of introducing an infection into the joint.

Stringhalt, Stifled, and Spavined

Let's talk about three afflictions of the hind leg: stringhalt, stifled, and spavined. These are horsemen's terms originating centuries ago that are easily confused and often poorly understood.

Stringhalt is a spastic overflexion of the hind leg. Usually only one leg is affected. As the horse lifts the leg to take a step it comes up too high, sometimes even hitting the belly, and then when the leg is returned to the ground, it does so with an exaggerated snap, the foot smartly slapping the ground. Stringhalt is seen in all breeds of horses. It tends to grow more severe with age. Most cases are worse when the horse is first led from the stall, and it then disappears as he is exercised. The stringhalt action is more obvious when the horse is turned sharply or backed up. It is also more of a problem in cold weather.

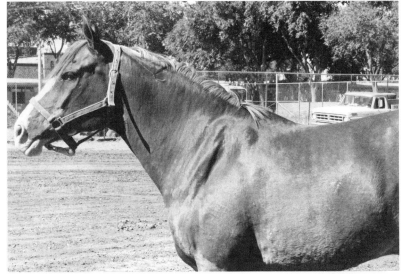

In the condition called sweeny, the shoulder muscles shrink, and the spine of the shoulder blade sticks out prominently.

The degree of abnormal action varies. Some horses are only mildly afflicted, showing just a slight overextension from which they quickly warm out. Such a horse can continue to be useful. I remember a good cowhorse I used to ride years ago that was stringhalted. He would warm out of the problem as soon as he had travelled a few hundred yards, and have no trouble the rest of the day. But on a cold morning, those first few yards were like riding a car with one tire blown out. Other cases can be so severe that the animal is useless as a saddle horse. *Any* horse that is stringhalted must be considered unsound.

The cause of stringhalt is not known. It may be due to neuritis of the sciatic or peroneal nerves, or possibly to a spinal cord lesion. There is no effective medicinal treatment. Most cases improve after surgical sectioning of one of the leg tendons, but only rarely does this produce a complete cure.

Sometimes a horse with a rope burn or wire cut in the back of the pastern will show a false stringhalt. A careful examination will reveal such an injury.

Stifled, though often confused with stringhalt, is an entirely different problem. The stifle joint of a horse corresponds to the human knee. It has a patella, or kneecap, at the front of the joint. Now some people say that a horse is stifled any time this joint is injured or unsound, but to me, the term refers to *dorsal patellar fixation.* By that I mean an upward dislocation of the kneecap. This condition is caused by a conformation fault, namely, a hind leg that is too straight. This is, therefore, an *inheritable* factor, and certain stallions are notorious for siring stifled foals. Although stifled horses may be seen in all breeds, Shetland ponies are particularly susceptible.

When the patella slips out of place, the hind leg locks in an extended position behind the body. In mild cases this is just momentary and the leg seems to "pop" or "catch" for a second. More severe cases may have the leg locked for several seconds, and the worst cases stay locked and are sometimes very difficult to put back in place.

The stifled foal will often outgrow his problem, especially if it is mild. But if it persists, or is severe, surgery is required. Delaying surgery beyond the age of three may leave the horse with a permanent gonitis (inflamed stifle joint). The operation is known as a medial patellar desmotomy. It is a simple operation, requiring just a few minutes to perform, and may be done under local anesthesia with the horse in a standing position. During the operation, a ligament is cut. When it heals, the ligament is longer than it originally was, thus preventing dislocation of the patella. The results are nearly always satisfactory. Most cases are completely normal after surgery.

Remember that there are many other stifle problems that can, to the untrained person, be confused with true dorsal patellar fixation.

Spavin is a disease of the hock joint.

There are several kinds of spavin, most of them characterized by a swelling in the hock region.

Blood spavin refers to an enlargement or varicosity of the saphenous vein. This blood vessel angles across the front of the hock joint. It is frequently associated with a bog spavin, which will be discussed next. A blood spavin may be considered a blemish rather than an unsoundness.

A *bog spavin* is a fluid-filled distension of the hock joint. When a horse has a bog spavin, the joint capsule of the hock stretches due to the excessive joint fluid being formed, and a bulge can be seen at the front of the hock.

The bulge is fluctuant. That is, if it is pressed, it does not feel hard, like bone, but is resilient. You can feel that it is filled with fluid. Usually additional bulges can be seen on the inside and/or the outside of the hock. These, too, will be fluctuant because the hock joint is extensive, and these pockets of fluid communicate with the bulge seen in front.

The fluid in a bog spavin is simply synovial fluid—a clear slippery liquid that serves as a joint lubricant (see the discussion of synovial effusion).

Bog spavins are most common in young, immature horses, and may be caused by a nutritional imbalance, a conformation defect, or a strain. In my opinion, most bog spavins in young horses (weanlings to three-year-olds) are simply due to strains. The excessive joint fluid, called a synovial effusion, is just a response of specialized synovial cells to injury.

I personally do not rely on conservative therapy when I treat a bog spavin. Rest, heat, liniments, or similar conservative treatments usually fail to stop the effusion. If the joint capsule becomes permanently stretched, the horse may not be lame, but will certainly be permanently blemished.

I find that if a bog spavin is attacked vigorously, and *early* (within a week or preferably less), in most cases the hock will look normal afterwards. Neglected cases tend to remain distended.

Bog spavins in young, growing horses should be radiographed (X-rayed) in order to rule out the presence of certain degenerative developmental joint dis-

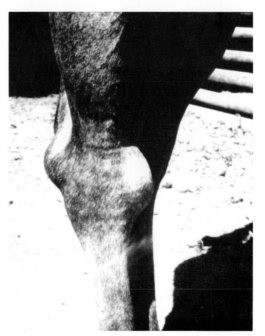

A bog spavin is a fluid-filled distension of the hock joint.

**Photo Courtesy of
Colorado State University**

eases, such as osteochondritis dessicans, often called "OCD." This is especially true if the bog spavin is accompanied by a limp involving the affected leg, or if a positive spavin test is obtained. A spavin test involves holding the hock in full flexion for a minute, and then trotting the horse out. A normal horse will trot out sound. If the horse limps on the tested limb, especially for the first several steps, we consider that to be a positive spavin test.

If the radiographic study is normal, and the horse simply has an uncomplicated bog, then I do the following treatment, which has, for me, been extremely satisfactory for many years.

I shave and surgically scrub that part of the hock that will permit access to the interior of the joint. If necessary, I sedate the horse. A thorough cleansing and disinfection of the skin is vital, because if infection of the joint develops, it is usually disastrous.

I then insert a needle into the joint space, and drain all of the fluid possible. I inspect this fluid, and in some cases send a sample off for laboratory analysis.

Then, I inject into the joint a mixture of a long-acting corticosteroid (a cortisone-type drug) and Depo-Provera (UpJohn).

Depo-Provera is a sex hormone, and ordinarily it is used intramuscularly in mares to delay estrus, or to maintain pregnancy. It is a long-acting progesterone. The reason I use such a surprising drug inside a joint, to treat a synovial effusion like bog spavin, is that Depo-Provera has anti-transudative properties. That is, it inhibits fluid formation within the joint capsule.

A word of caution: This drug should not be used in mares that will soon be bred because, as the hormone is absorbed from the joint space into the system, it will interfere with the heat cycle.

After the injection is complete, the hock may be bandaged with a pressure-type dressing, although I often do not do this.

For a few days, the hock may look as full as ever. Then, in most cases, if the bog spavin has not been there too long, it goes away.

This technique is effective when the bog spavin is recent and has been caused by strain. When the bog is caused by poor conformation or a nutritional imbalance, the effusion will usually recur despite the treatment.

I always give a patient a full month of rest after such an injection. That is *very* important. The horse should be kept in a stall for at least a few days. Then, if the bog spavin was not too severe, the horse can have access to a corral. When training is resumed, it should be done very gradually.

Occasionally, this treatment fails to remove a bog—usually because it has been present too long (weeks or months). In such a case, I will attempt a second treatment after 30 days. However, if the first treatment fails, a second will rarely work. When a bog is first seen, it is extremely important to start treatment as soon as possible, and then to allow a long rest period.

Bone spavin is the worst type of spavin. It is an arthritic lesion of the hock joint, often associated with conformation faults that increase concussion in the hock. Most bone spavins are caused by strain and injury as for example in calf roping, when horses are subjected to severe sliding stops. If calf roping horses are properly fed, kept free of worms, selected for perfect hind limb conformation, and not started at roping calves until at least four years of age, then spavin is much less likely to develop.

Bone spavin causes stubborn lameness. Veterinary examination and X-ray studies will confirm the diagnosis. Most cases show a bony enlargement on the inner side of the hock, often called a *jack* by horsemen.

A bone spavin is incurable, but several treatments may keep the horse serviceable. Corrective shoeing with a special spavin shoe helps some horses. Surgical removal of part of the cunean tendon may give relief when the spavin lies under that tendon. Pain may be eliminated by fusing the involved bones by cautery or surgery. Surgical fusion (arthrodesis) of the joint, developed by Dr. O.R. Adams, has been especially successful. Sometimes the veterinarian will combine two or even all three methods. Diathermy, X-ray therapy, or ultrasound treatments combined with rest have also been used in mild cases. Anti-inflammatory and pain-relieving drugs

117

are often helpful in managing the disease.

An *occult* or *blind spavin* involves the joint surfaces of the hock and shows no jack or bony enlargement. In fact, X-ray studies sometimes fail to reveal the lesion. Occult spavin is treated much the same way as an ordinary spavin. Both jacks and occult spavins are serious and can cause permanent unsoundnesses in the horse.

Bursitis

Bursitis is a disease that occurs more often in the horse than in any other domestic animal. A bursitis is an inflamed bursa. Well now, what is a bursa? The word means purse in Latin, and that's what a bursa is—a small purse or sack. These sacks are found in various parts of the body, filled with a slippery lubricating fluid, and they serve to protect prominent bony places and where tendons play over bone. When a bursa is injured, it swells, becomes hot and painful, and the amount of fluid in it becomes greatly increased. In horses, simple bursitis often becomes complicated with infection. The infected bursa then breaks and drains, and may form a fistula that refuses to heal.

If you have been a horseman for any length of time, you are quite familiar with several types of bursitis. For example, *fistula of the withers* is an infected bursitis of the bursa on top of the backbone in the region of the withers. *Poll evil* is an infected bursitis of a bursa located on top of the head. A *shoe boil* is bursitis of the elbow. *Capped hock* refers to a bursitis at the point of the hock. A bursitis at the pin bones—those bony prominences of the rump—is known as a *car bruise.* There is a bursa deep in the foot where a tendon plays over the navicular sesamoid bone. Such a bursitis is called *navicular disease,* and ultimately the inflammation eats into the bone itself. Up in the hip region the trochanteric bursa may flare up to cause *whorlbone lameness.* And, there is a shoulder lameness caused by *intertubercular bursitis.*

Why are horses, more than other animals, so prone to bursitis? Well, the horse is an athlete. Using him as we do subjects his body to many strains. If a cow were ridden, jumped, whirled, run, and banged around as is a horse, she would undoubtedly suffer more bursitis than she does. You see, a bursa becomes inflamed and swollen from injury. The injury might be a sudden severe one, such as a horse bumping the top of his head on a doorway and ending up with poll evil, but more often the injury is slight and endlessly repeated. A horse could develop bursitis of the withers from rolling on a stone, but usually it comes from constant injury to the withers from an ill-fitting saddle.

What can you do to prevent bursitis in your horses? Prevent injury! See that the doorway is high enough so that your horse won't bump his head. Ride a saddle that fits the horse's back, with the fork high enough to clear the withers. Use thick, good quality, and clean saddle blankets and pads. If you rope heavy cattle, use the thickest felt pads you can find.

Capped hocks nowadays are most often due to bruising them against the tailgate of a trailer. Pad the hocks, or the tailgate, or both if possible. Shoe boil is caused from pressure on the elbow bursa by the heel of a shoe. Such pressure may occur when the horse lies down with his legs tucked under him. Or, the shoe may repeatedly strike the elbow when the horse stamps at flies. Fly spray will solve the latter problem, while a shoe boil ring will take care of the former. A shoe boil ring is a doughnut-like cushion that is worn around the pastern to prevent pressure of the heel on the point of the elbow.

Navicular disease is partially a conformation problem. That is, it is more common in horses with a poor shock-absorbing system—poor conformation. However, since concussion is the cause, it is common sense to limit riding a horse on hard surfaces. Also, a light shoe does not absorb concussion as well as a heavier shoe with a wider web. Trimming the foot too low at the heel puts greater pressure on the navicular bursa, so proper foot care also helps to prevent this type of bursitis.

Naturally, despite the best of care, some horses will still develop some type of bursitis. Like most diseases, a cure depends on a prompt and accurate diagnosis, followed by effective treatment. Sometimes the diagnosis of a disease is simple, as in an obvious shoe boil or capped hock. At other times, as in navicular disease or intertubercular bursitis, the veterinarian may have to use some elaborate techniques to confirm the diagnosis. Manipulation, careful observation, X-ray pictures, and nerve blocking may be necessary to prove some kinds of bursitis.

The treatment of a diseased bursa will vary with the length of time the condition is present, where it is located in the body, and whether infection is present. Surgery is often necessary. Other cases will respond to antibiotics, or cortisone drugs, or chemical therapy.

It is *always* necessary to rest the part, and to remove the *cause* that damaged the bursa. Some cases, such as an old chronic case of navicular disease, are incurable.

The diagnosis and treatment of bursal lesions are the veterinarian's problem. As a horseman, your problem is one of prevention. Go back and reread the various kinds of bursitis we have enumerated. Think about the cause of each kind. What rules of good horsemanship are you neglecting that may ultimately lead to a disfiguring or crippling bursitis?

Synovial Effusion

The living body has many moving parts. Like any piece of machinery, lubrication is necessary to prevent excessive friction and wear of these parts, and to ensure smooth operation. To do this, the body manufactures a lubricant called *synovia.*

Synovia is a slick, smooth, yellowish fluid. You may think of it as "joint oil." Wherever lubrication is needed, certain specialized cells form this oil. Every joint is lined with such cells. We call this lining a synovial membrane. In the joint, the membrane constantly manufactures small amounts of synovia to ease the motion of the joint—just as oil does a hinge. If the oil were absent, the joint would soon "rust," and become corroded and creaky. The entire joint, which is surrounded by a leak-proof capsule, is filled with synovia.

Other parts of the body are also lined with synovial membrane. The tendons that operate the joints are simply cables.

These cables run through a flexible tubing that is lubricated with synovia. All over the body, at points of wear and tear, are little lubricating sacks called *bursa.* Inside the bursa is, again, a synovial membrane. The synovia inside the bursa acts as a water cushion against concussion, bumps, and friction.

When a part of the body containing a synovial membrane is injured, inflammation sets in. This means that heat, swelling, and pain occur. The blood vessels in the inflamed area dilate, so more blood moves to this area.

If the inflammation is in a joint, we call it *arthritis.* If it is in a bursa, we refer to it as *bursitis.* And if in a tendon sheath, we say *tenosynovitis,* or bowed tendon. These conditions can occur in humans as well as in horses and other animals.

The injury that causes the inflammation might be a sudden, severe one. For example, a horse's knee might be struck by a polo mallet. An acute arthritis of the knee follows. Or, the injury might be a slight, repeated one. As an example, the heel of the shoe may continuously bruise the point of the elbow when the horse lies down, or stamps at flies. There is a bursa at the point of the elbow, and inflammation of this bursa produces the familiar "shoe boil."

Due to the heat and increased blood supply, the synovial membrane is stimulated to produce more synovia than is ordinarily needed to lubricate the part. Therefore, the synovial sac starts to swell with an accumulation of excess synovia. That's why the polo pony's knee balloons up with "water on the knee." Or, the injured bursa at the point of the elbow fills with synovia. The fluid inside of a shoe boil is simple synovia.

This excessive outpouring of synovia is called, technically, a *synovial effusion.* A great number of common ailments in the horse, with mysterious and ancient names, are nothing more than synovial effusion. These include water on the knee, shoe boil, capped hock, wind puffs or wind gall, thoroughpin, bog spavin, whorlbone lameness, and tendon galls.

Synovial effusion is also part of the problems involved in poll evil, fistula of the withers, navicular disease, bowed tendon, popped knee, and all kinds of joint diseases.

What happens if a synovial effusion is not treated? Well, the body, of course, is capable of healing many injuries without help. Providing that the part is *rested*, nature alone may repair the injury. As inflammation subsides, the excessive secretion of synovia slows down. The fluid is absorbed by the body. The swelling in the injured area subsides.

Sometimes the capsule surrounding the part is so stretched that it can never completely shrink to where it was before. It remains permanently distended. This is what happens in a bog spavin, a wind puff, or a thoroughpin. Such a swelling may be unsightly, but might not cause future trouble. It is considered to be a blemish, rather than an unsoundness. We might point out here that conformation faults, or inheritable defects, may weaken a part so that it is more susceptible to injury, and hence to synovial effusion. But the effusion itself is caused by injury, either sudden and severe, or repeated and mild, as pointed out before.

Sometimes bacteria gain entrance to the synovial accumulation, and infection then sets in. This is what happens in poll evil, or fistula of the withers. A simple bursitis becomes infected, causing a very serious problem indeed.

And, unfortunately, sometimes nature fails completely, and the synovial effusion becomes chronic. The synovial membrane grows thicker. More and more synovia is produced. The part becomes more swollen and pressure increases. Finally, scar tissue starts to build up, and in time, calcium deposits are laid down. The horse that originally had a swollen water-filled knee now has a great knob of rock-hard calcium. The joint can no longer bend. The horse is ruined. The horse with the shoe boil has a chronic, disfiguring cystic mass for which no treatment is effective except radical surgery to remove the entire elbow bursa. Uncontrolled chronic synovial effusion leads to crippling permanent arthritis, tendon deformity, and disfiguring chronic capped hocks, elbows, and knees. This is the reason that every synovial effusion should be treated at once!

What can be done to stop a synovial effusion? First of all, the part must be rested. The horse must immediately stop work completely. Second, the part involved should be examined by a veterinarian to determine the cause of the effusion. Is the big knee due to a blow, a strain, or a fracture? Is the lump on the withers caused by an ill-fitting saddle? Is the bog or thoroughpin the result of overworking a young horse, or poor conformation? Third, treatment must be started at once to subdue the effusion.

Using the most careful, sterile technique to avoid infection, we drain the excessive synovia from the part. This will help prevent permanent stretching and distension of the capsule. Next, we inject powerful anti-inflammatory drugs *into* the synovial cavity. These drugs act directly on the synovial membrane, relieving the heat, pain, and excessive circulation, and thereby discourage the membrane from producing so much synovia. This treatment is repeated as often as is necessary. If the part is superficial, ice packs will help to cool it and lessen the amount of synovia being produced. This anti-inflammatory treatment must be continued until the synovial effusion is completely quenched.

Meanwhile, the horse must be rested. The injury that caused the effusion must be stopped. If the part is in the legs, no exercise is permitted. If it is a shoe boil, a special padded shoe boil ring is put around the pastern to prevent further injury by the heel of the shoe. Capped hocks must be protected by sponge rubber pads. The rest must continue long after the effusion is stopped to permit complete healing. Remember that this treatment stops the effusion. It does not heal the injury that caused the effusion in the first place. Only time and nature can do that.

Remember, too, that this treatment must be started immediately if you want good results. Every day that it is delayed means a poorer chance of recovery. Once the synovial membrane has become chronically thickened, scarred, and calcified, nothing will help except radical surgery of one kind or another. And, while some parts may be reached surgically with little difficulty, other parts may not. A chronic cap on the hock isn't difficult to remove. But a stifle joint with a synovial effusion of two years' duration cannot be operated on.

So don't be confused with the myriad

horsemen's terms—the puffs, galls, boils, and thoroughpins. These swellings are all caused by excessive secretion of synovia: plain ol' joint oil. Remember that synovial effusion *can* be stopped by modern drugs, but that drugs must be used as soon as possible for satisfactory results. Understand that, treated or not, rest is absolutely essential for proper healing of the part. Remember that a neglected synovial effusion might mean a permanent blemish, or the ruin of the horse.

Knee Injuries

The knee of the horse is not really a knee. This important joint of the front leg is properly called the *carpus,* and it corresponds, anatomically, to the human wrist. Remember that we are discussing the horse's *front* leg, which is similar to our own arm. In the hind leg, it is the stifle joint of the horse that corresponds to the human knee.

Be that as it may, horsemen everywhere call the equine carpus a knee, so a knee it shall remain.

This part of the horse's leg is frequently injured. The knee hits jumps, bumps posts and mangers, is often bruised by the great weight of the horse when he slips and falls. The knee joint, like our own wrist, is composed of many small bones. Therefore, it is not a highly stable joint, structurally speaking, and it is readily injured. Severe strains or blows can easily fracture one of the small knee bones. And a high splint sometimes invades the knee joint.

When a horse injures his knee, the first thing I recommend is an ice pack. When I speak of injury, I do not include those injuries involving a break in the skin. (Penetrating wounds of *any* joint should have prompt professional attention.) I mean injuries in which the knee is hurt, but the skin is not broken.

The ice pack, used repeatedly over a 24-hour period, and an elastic bandage (not too tight) will often prevent the knee from "blowing up" or developing "water on the knee." Many bruised knees will be normal after a day of icing.

Do *not* apply heat or liniment right after the injury occurs. Heat will only further inflame an already-inflamed area. If there is bleeding within the knee, ice packs will tend to stop the bleeding as well as reduce pain, swelling, and inflammation.

If, after this initial therapy, the knee is not normal, call your veterinarian.

Whenever there is marked lameness and distension, I believe that the horse should be X-rayed to rule out a fracture. When taking such X-rays, multiple views at various angles are necessary because small carpal fractures are often not visible on an X-ray unless seen exactly from the right angle. Many such fractures require surgery if the horse is to have a chance of regaining soundness.

When a knee is swollen, warm, and filled with fluid, it does not necessarily mean that the joint itself is injured. You'll notice that with many such knees, the horse is not lame. In such a knee, a bursa, under the skin, fills with fluid. It is important that such a bursa be promptly drained and injected with the proper medication. If it is neglected, the swelling becomes cystic and will require surgery to reduce it. If nothing is done, this cystic mass, called a "hygroma," will eventually calcify—and the horse is permanently blemished and the knee flexion is impaired.

You have, perhaps, heard the term "popped knee." This term is usually used when an acute carpitis (arthritis of the knee due to an injury) is present. This is a serious injury that can leave a horse permanently unsound.

To summarize, when a horse injures a knee, ice-pack it the first day. If it is not normal the next day, call a veterinarian. Using home remedies a week or two before calling the veterinarian might greatly interfere with his ability to restore the horse to normal.

Bowed Tendons

Look at one of your horse's legs. At the back of the cannon bone you can see and feel the great flexor tendons that are sometimes called cords or leaders by horsemen. These tendons are attached down low at the hoof.

They act as cables, connecting the muscles at the back of the forearm with the hoof. When these muscles contract, the hoof flexes—just as your own forearm muscles flex your fingers.

There are actually two tendons, with

If there is bleeding within the knee, ice packs will tend to stop the bleeding as well as reduce pain, swelling, and inflammation.

121

A bowed tendon is caused by strain. It can happen when the tendon is stressed beyond its endurance in a long race or at extreme speed.

one overlying the other, at the back of the horse's cannon. They are called the deep and superficial digital flexor tendons. The tendons are covered with a sheath that is lubricated with synovia, a natural body fluid.

When an injury occurs to these tendons and their sheath, causing bleeding and a tearing of the tendon fibers or the tendon sheath, we say that the tendon has bowed. A bowed tendon is very painful, hot, and swollen. The horse with a bowed tendon will never be the same. But, with proper care the damage can be minimized, and the horse's chances for continued usefulness will be enhanced.

A bowed tendon is caused by strain. It can happen when the tendon is stressed beyond its endurance in a long race or at extreme speed. A horse that is not in good physical condition—i.e., a *soft* horse—can easily bow a tendon while loping uphill, while bucking, or as the result of sudden acceleration or a hard turn. A severe blow to the tendon can also cause damage resulting in a bowed tendon.

Although there are different ways to treat a bowed tendon, almost all veterinarians agree that the following points are important:

1/ A bowed tendon is a serious injury that can ruin a horse.

2/ A bowed tendon must be treated at once. Any delay will reduce the chances for optimum healing.

3/ Even after it is healed, a bowed tendon will never again be as strong as it was originally.

4/ It takes a *full* year for the tendon to heal completely, regardless of the method of treatment.

This last point is very important. Too often the owner's impatience interferes with proper repair. Remember that even though the injury seems to be healed after a few weeks, it will be a year before *complete* healing takes place. A horse with a bowed tendon *must* be laid up and rested.

Before I discuss the treatment of a bowed tendon, I should talk about some conditions that resemble a bow:

First of all, the term "bow" is not a scientific medical term, but a horseman's term that simply describes the bulging or bowing of the flexor tendon when

viewed from the side. In other words, the tendon is *swollen*.

The reader should realize that swelling can occur without actual damage to the tendon structure. For example, bandaging a leg too tightly can cause damage to the tendon area with subsequent swelling, causing the tendon to *look* bowed. Most of the time, the damage from a tight bandage is superficial, involving only the skin, the subcutaneous tissues, and sometimes the tendon sheath. Usually the tendon itself is not damaged, and that means that the recovery will be faster than if there is actual tendon damage. However, a tight bandage, left on long enough, *can* cause true tendon damage. Theoretically, if a bandage is tight enough to cut circulation, the entire leg can be lost, so beware the tight bandage.

Other swellings that resemble a bow can result from a bruise to the back of the leg. This can occur from over-reaching, or from banging the back of the leg on a rail or the top of a stall door, or from a kick by another horse. Infections, too, especially of the tendon sheath, will resemble a bowed tendon.

You can see why a swollen tendon should be seen promptly by a competent equine practitioner. Once the proper diagnosis is made, appropriate treatment can be selected.

For many years I have used the following treatment for bowed tendons with extremely pleasing results. It is not the *only* way to treat a bow, but this method has worked wonderfully well for me.

1/ As soon as the bow is detected, I pack the leg in ice water. A light pressure bandage is applied. The first aid will help stop the bleeding within the tendon sheath, and minimize pain and swelling. I like to ice the leg for about 24 hours.

2/ The next day I drain any accumulation of fluid or blood. If none can be drained, I apply wet dressings of a diluted DMSO compound for a day or so. Then I treat the horse with corticosteroids systemically. Sometimes I inject the steroids right into the tendon.

3/ The horse is confined to a stall. Absolute rest is essential. I immobilize the leg with a light cast. The leg is checked every week or two, and treatment may be repeated as indicated.

4/ After the cast is removed, the horse

is laid up for rest for six to twelve months, preferably twelve. A small corral or paddock is ideal for the first few months. Later, a larger corral or pasture may be used if available.

In western saddle horses with bowed tendons, the great majority treated this way will remain serviceably sound.

Some very severe bows may require surgical treatment. These bows are most often seen on the racetrack. In pleasure and show horse practice, bows this severe don't occur too often. However, there is an exception to this statement and that is the "low bow." A bow involving the flexor tendon just above the fetlock can be very serious, even if the swelling is relatively slight. The tendon in that area is bound by a structure called the annular ligament, and bows under that ligament are particularly serious. Sometimes, even long after the tendon has healed, the annular ligament must be cut to relieve pressure on the permanently thickened tendon. Such an operation is called an annular desmotomy. Desmotomy means "ligament cutting."

Even slight bows heal with permanent thickening and scarring of the tendon, which are obvious to the experienced veterinarian when he feels the tendon.

Once again, if enough time is given for complete healing, *most* horses with bowed tendons can be returned to service, even though the tendon is deformed in its appearance, and has lost its original elasticity.

Putting the injured horse back to work too soon is an invitation to chronic tendinitis—a tendon that is always more or less sore—and a horse that cannot perform soundly.

After a bowed tendon is well on its way to healing (many weeks), I like to prescribe physical therapy. This may involve a special shoe, but always involves heat therapy. I find that the most effective use of ultrasound is in the treatment of healing bowed tendons, but other forms of heat are also very helpful. These include diathermy, a warm jacuzzi, moist heating pads, etc. The choice of physical therapy will vary with the personal preference and experience of the veterinarian. Chemical blisters are popular because they are simple to apply, but I don't think they are as effective as the more penetrating methods mentioned above.

The biggest problem, I have found, is persuading the owner to be patient and rest the horse long enough. This treatment can be so spectacularly effective that the rider will be tempted to start using the horse too soon. Never gamble a horse's entire future for a few months of use. When a veterinarian lays a horse up for a prescribed length of time, make up your mind to follow his instructions.

Foot Problems

The horse's foot is a complex structure. It has a bony core at the center, known as the coffin bone. Outside, it is covered with hard protective hoof. Between these two firm structures lies an involved mechanism of soft structures that serve to nourish the foot, support the great weight above it, and act as shock absorbers and springs. There are blood vessels and nerves, a spongy fibrous cushion, ligaments and lubricating bursae, supporting wings of cartilage, sensitive membranes, and even a special layer of cells that secrete periople—the "shellac" that naturally covers the hoof wall.

Such a complicated piece of machinery is bound to break down at times, especially when one considers the pounding and punishment it must endure. We have, in other discussions, described several diseases of the foot, including navicular disease and founder. Now we shall consider several more common diseases of the equine foot.

Thrush. This is a disease of the frog of the foot characterized by decomposition of the hoof material and resultant infection. It is the result of excessive moisture, filth, and lack of air. Thrush usually begins in the grooves of the frog, and in advanced cases may destroy the entire frog. The horse may not show lameness or pain unless the case is well-advanced. Thrush is easily recognized by its foul odor and thick, wet, black discharge. Contracted feet with atrophied, sunken frogs are especially prone to thrush.

Fortunately, most cases of thrush are fairly easy to cure. The horse must be moved to clean, dry surroundings. The diseased tissue should be trimmed away,

Big, painful sidebones are usually the result of chronic injury due to concussion and hard traveling.

and the foot cleaned daily. The infection may be destroyed with antibiotics, sulfa drugs, germicides, and various lotions. Frankly, most cases will clear up spontaneously if the foot is properly cleaned up and *kept* clean. Occasional cases prove very stubborn. Severe cases in which the frog has been destroyed may require corrective shoeing. A bar shoe will help relieve contracted heels.

Quarter cracks. Cracks in the hoof originating at the coronet band and proceeding down the hoof wall are called sand cracks or quarter cracks. If the crack is at the toe, it is called a toe crack. Deep cracks open wider when the horse steps on the foot. They may bleed and often become infected and very painful. Dry brittle hoofs are prone to crack. Prompt treatment is important to stop the progress of a crack. We do this in several ways, depending on the location and depth of the crack, and whether infection is present. The methods used include grooving of the hoof, corrective shoeing, plastic repair of the defect, clinching the crack, and sometimes cautery. Infections are treated with disinfectants, new hoof growth is encouraged by applying stimulants to the coronet, and the hoof is made supple by applying hoof dressings.

Cracks can be avoided by good foot care. This means regular trimming and shoeing. The outside wall of the hoof should not be rasped because this removes the natural protective periople.

Dry feet should be dressed often with a hoof dressing. I personally don't think the particular formula makes much difference so long as it doesn't contain harmful chemicals—as does, for example, crankcase oil. Oils, waxes, and greases all serve to coat the hoof, thereby limiting the escape of natural moisture that is already in the hoof. Any vegetable or animal oil, fat, or wax compound will do (paraffin, beeswax, lanolin, Neatsfoot oil, bacon fat, etc.).

Contracted heels. Contraction of the heels is not a disease. It is a symptom of poor shoeing, or pain. Pain, such as is present in navicular disease or chronic corns, or other foot disorders, will cause the horse to bear less weight on the foot. When an organ is not used, it atrophies. So does the foot. As the foot atrophies, the heel contracts.

Sidebones. When the flexible, springy, lateral cartilages of the horse's foot turn to bone, we refer to them as sidebones. In some horses, especially big, heavy individuals, this process occurs rather normally as they age. If sidebones cause no lameness, they are best ignored. However, sidebones can and do cause lameness in many horses. Big, painful sidebones are usually the result of chronic injury due to concussion and hard traveling. Barbed wire cuts into the lateral cartilage area often result in sidebone formation after a few years.

Painful sidebones may be relieved by corrective shoeing and foot trimming, and by the use of various drugs. Before prescribing a corrective shoe or other therapy for sidebone, the veterinarian will often order X-ray studies of the foot to rule out other complicating causes of lameness, and to determine the extent of the sidebone.

These are just a few of the many foot disorders that affect the horse. A complete list would have to include founder, canker, grease heel, bruised sole, abscessed sole, quittor, seedy toe, keratoma, navicular disease, fracture of the coffin bone, pedal osteitis, pyramidal disease, coronet bruises, abscesses of the coronet, navicular fracture, heel injuries due to over-reaching, pumice foot, and many others.

There's a lot to know, isn't there? The correction of these problems is a job for the farrier and veterinarian. Your concern as a horse owner is to prevent these foot problems.

In the few conditions we discussed, you may have noticed that proper foot care was mentioned as a requisite for preventing trouble. Once again, good management and proper horse husbandry are the best ways to avoid trouble. The same is true of most of the other foot diseases we named. Most of them are preventable if you observe the basic rules of horsemanship.

Take care of your horse's feet. Keep them clean. Try to find a reliable, competent horseshoer. He should see your horse every six weeks. Keep those feet well-trimmed, well-shod, and dress them if they are dry and brittle. Don't ride on pavement unnecessarily, and then don't go faster than a walk. Pick out the sole often. Examine the feet daily, especially

124

before you ride. When an injury occurs, don't neglect it. And don't just take care of the feet. Take care of the whole horse. He's not much use to you if you can't ride him, and you can't ride him if he's lame.

Poor shoeing, leaving shoes on too long, or foolishly trimming away the frog, will cause the heels to contract. The mechanism of the foot causes the heels to spread when pressure is applied to the frog. If the frog is lacking, or if the foot has grown so long that the frog cannot touch the ground, the heels will contract.

To correct contracted heels, remove the source of pain, if one exists and it is removable. Then apply corrective care. Mild cases may be relieved by simple frog pressure. This may be accomplished by traveling barefoot on a full frog. If the horse must be shod, a bar shoe may be made, providing frog pressure. Severe cases require very special shoeing at frequent intervals, plus grooving of the hoof wall. Keep the foot well-covered with a hoof dressing.

Corns. In horses, corns are most often caused by a bruising of the sole at the junction of the wall and the bar of the foot. Such bruising can be caused by pressure of an ill-fitting shoe heel, or improper trimming. If neglected, a corn may become infected, thus leading to serious complications. To correct a corn, the foot must be carefully trimmed and skillfully shod. Infected corns require surgical drainage.

Puncture wounds. Horses often puncture the sole by stepping on nails, rakes, or other sharp objects. Do not delay when this occurs. Prompt veterinary attention may prevent a case of tetanus, or a severely abscessed foot. Waiting a day or two to see what happens can be terribly costly when a foot is punctured.

Navicular Disease

One of the most common and serious causes of lameness in saddle horses is navicular disease. The navicular bone is a small, flat, elliptical bone that lies in back of the coffin joint, down inside the heel of the foot. It is a sesamoid bone, serving as a sort of pulley over which runs the big flexor tendon just before it attaches to the coffin bone.

Between the navicular bone and the tendon is a bursa or lubricating sack. Navicular disease begins with an inflammation of this bursa, caused by strain of one kind or another. In other words, the problem begins with a navicular bursitis. As the months and years go by, the inflammation extends from the bursa to the adjacent bone and often to the attachment of the tendon. The bone, once involved, progressively degenerates, and the horse grows lamer as time goes on.

Navicular disease can involve any of the four feet, but is most common in the front feet. Often both forefeet are involved, but one will be worse, giving the impression that there is lameness only in that foot. We see navicular disease in all breeds of horses, and at all ages, although it most frequently appears at six to nine years of age.

Usually navicular disease appears first as a mild, recurrent, and insidious lameness. It may take years for the classical symptoms to appear. These include limping, especially when first moved out, pointing of the involved feet in an attempt to relieve pressure on the painful heel, a choppy characteristic gait, stumbling, and progressive changes in the appearance of the foot. The chronic navicular disease foot is atrophied, narrow, contracted, brittle, high at the heel, with an arched sole and shrunken frog. If the opposing foot is normal, or at least more normal, the diseased foot will be distinctly smaller in size.

Of course, these symptoms are also typical of other kinds of lameness. In order to confirm his diagnosis, the veterinarian will resort to diagnostic nerve blocking, and X-ray pictures.

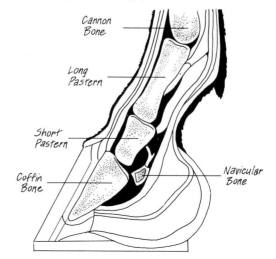

Cannon Bone

Long Pastern

Short Pastern

Coffin Bone

Navicular Bone

Navicular disease is incurable, but several kinds of treatment are available to relieve pain and thereby extend the useful life of the horse. These include: corrective shoeing, pain-relieving drugs, and neurectomy. The neurectomy is a surgical operation wherein the nerves back in the heel area are severed. All of these treatments are only of temporary value and the owner of the horse must realize that if a horse with navicular disease continues to work, that the disease will be aggravated and its progress hastened.

Neurectomy

The term "nerving" is familiar to most experienced horse owners. Or, we may hear that a horse is "nerved" or has had a "nerving" operation. These terms refer to a surgical procedure known as *neurectomy*, wherein certain nerves are severed for the relief of lameness, when all else fails.

Obviously, cutting the nerve that provides a part of the body with feeling may relieve pain, but it does nothing to otherwise affect the disease process that is causing the pain. In fact, because the horse that is successfully neurectomized will stop favoring the involved limb, and use it more fully, neurectomy may actually worsen the disease process. Nevertheless, this is a valuable and justifiable operation in certain cases.

Actually, any part of the horse's leg may be nerved. Theoretically, it is possible to entirely deaden a horse's leg by cutting the proper nerves, but by far the most common application for neurectomy involves the nerves that supply the heel. The most common *reason* for deadening the heels is to relieve the pain of navicular disease (see the discussions of navicular disease and on diagnostic nerve blocking).

In most states, horses that have had heel nerving are allowed to race, and a horse so operated is still safe to ride because it still has feeling in the balance of the foot. However, because the heels are numbed, such a horse may step on a nail that penetrates the heel, or otherwise injure the back part of the foot, and will not feel it or indicate the injury by limping. So the owner of the horse may not be aware of such a wound until infection

sets in. Therefore, the feet of a nerved horse must be inspected often.

Sometimes the nerves supplying the rest of the foot, or the ankle, or even the upper portions of the leg are nerved, but this is more dangerous than just doing the heel area. The horse with an entirely dead foot cannot feel the ground, and is more likely to stumble or fall. There is also a complication of nerving that sometimes occurs, and that is that the hoof may slough (rot off). This rarely happens when the heel alone is nerved, but is more likely to occur if higher nerves are cut.

One form of neurectomy, involving the median nerve up in the forearm, is controversial. It is frowned on, in general, in the United States, because it deadens so much of the leg, yet, in some European countries, it is commonly done for lameness originating higher in the leg, as in the knee. I have never personally done a median neurectomy, but I have seen a number of horses that have had the operation and that continued to perform safely and effectively (steer roping, jumping, etc.). So, I'm not sure that this operation shouldn't be more widely accepted and more frequently performed. Advocates of median neurectomy claim that the horse is left with enough feeling in its leg to perform safely. This controversy would make a good university research project.

Before neurectomy is performed, the owner should realize these things:

1/ In general, the procedure should be regarded as a last resort, when more conservative measures have failed. In navicular disease, for example, most patients can be kept going with corrective shoeing and with medications, for a long time—sometimes for years—before neurectomy is necessary.

2/ The results of neurectomy are not predictable and are not 100 percent effective. For example, about 50 percent of all horses have extra nerve branches supplying the heel. In such cases the relief of pain may be partial rather than complete. Failures can occur.

3/ Neurectomy is rarely permanent. Nerves do try to regrow, and even with the best surgical techniques, the horse may go lame again in the future. Sometimes a tumor, called a *neuroma*, forms at the end of a cut nerve, and this can be more painful than the original condition. Neurectomized horses *can* sometimes be reoperated successfully if and when the original operation fails.

4/ Remember that cutting the nerves only relieves pain. It does not stop the condition causing the pain. So even if, for example, a heel nerving operation (posterior or palmar digital neurectomy) is completely successful for a horse with navicular disease, the disease process goes on. Sooner or later, even it it takes years, the disease may extend beyond the deadened area, so that lameness returns, or the disease will destroy vital structures, such as the flexor tendon, completely crippling the horse and necessitating humane destruction.

In spite of all the above disadvantages, neurectomy is a very valuable procedure for the relief of selected lameness problems. It stops pain and enables many fine performance horses to go on with their competitive career.

Ice

Wouldn't it be wonderful if there were a medicine that cost nothing, was available almost anywhere, was free of harmful side effects, could relieve pain, reduce swelling of acute injuries, prevent complications, and shorten healing time? Well, there is such a thing: ice.

The application of cold to acute injuries (*acute* means fresh or very recent), such as sprains, strains, and bruises, is of great value. How acute should the injury be? The sooner treatment is started, the more effective it will be.

To avoid misunderstanding, let's give some examples of the kind of injury we mean. We're not talking about wounds, such as lacerations or punctures with external bleeding, or major breaks in the skin. When we say "sprains, strains, and bruises," we refer to injuries of the musculo-skeletal system that are so common in horses. These include the sprained fetlock, the suspensory ligament sprain, the flexor tendon injury (bowed tendon), the bruised cannon or knee, the bruised hock (that will later fill, causing capped hock), the muscle hematoma that occurs when a horse is kicked in the shoulder or rump, or the bone bruise that occurs when a splint bone is struck by the opposite foot.

All of these injuries are characterized by trauma to soft tissues of the body such as ligaments, tendons, periosteum (the membrane that covers bone), muscles, and subcutaneous structures. When such an injury happens, blood vessels are ruptured and cells are damaged. Blood leaks out of the ruptured vessels, causing swelling and pain. Eventually the blood will clot, and separate into solid and liquid parts.

The liquid, called serum, takes a long time to absorb, and may accumulate to form pockets of liquid as in "water on the knee." The injured cells release chemicals that cause further pain, swelling, and heat. This combination of pain, swelling, and heat is known as inflammation, and rapid cooling of the injured part as soon as possible after the injury occurs will reduce inflammation. Ice is not the only way cold can be applied. Cold water from a hose (if it is cold enough) or a running stream are excellent. So are chemical cold packs, ice bags, and snow. Dry ice (solid carbon dioxide) should *not* be used because it is too cold, and will damage tissues by freezing them.

For the injured limb, immersion in a mixture of cracked ice and water for several hours is satisfactory. Treatment for less than an hour is going to be of minimal value.

For lower leg injuries, you can stand the horse in a bucket of ice water. If the injury is above the water level in the bucket, some horsemen improvise by standing the horse in a bucket, then wrapping a wet towel around the injury.

Or special boots are available (at tack stores) for soaking legs. You can also make your own boot by cutting an inner tube to make a long "sock," and sealing one end with glue or tying it off.

For head injuries, or injuries of upper body parts, an ice bag may be applied. A little ingenuity may be required.

Of course, if the injury is obviously severe or if it hasn't responded satisfactorily to initial icing, call your veterinarian. Remember that what looks like a simple bone bruise may be a fracture, and that many inflammations require more extensive treatment than just cooling. Remember, too, that an infection also is inflamed, and that cooling will not help if an infection is present.

MARES AND FOALS

Raising a foal is a considerable investment of money and time.

Breeding Decisions

This article may be of interest to you if you are thinking about raising a foal—especially if you are a novice at the game. Before breeding your mare you must ask yourself several questions:

1/ Why do I want to breed her? If you are breeding the mare because you think it will improve her physically or mentally, don't bother. Motherhood doesn't change a mare, and don't apply anthropomorphic ideas to an animal.

If you are breeding her for the experience of raising a foal, remember this: Although raising a foal *is* an experience, foals are cute little devils for only a few short weeks. Thereafter you can look forward to a couple of years of support-

Photo by Debbie Freitag

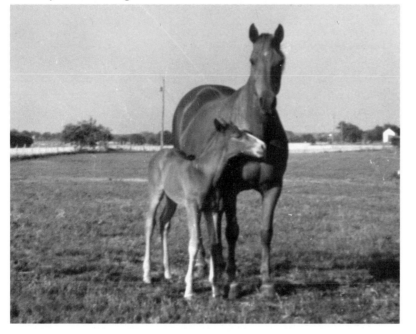

ing a grain and hay devouring youngster before he's old enough to break and ride.

If you are breeding your mare because you need another horse, don't overlook what the horse is going to cost you.

Years will go by before you can ride that foal. During this time you will have many expenses. There will be stud fees, transportation costs, veterinary bills, extra feed for the mare, bedding, and foot trimming bills for the foal. These costs plus feeding your growing foal will add up fast. Now stop and think of the kind of horse, ready to ride, that you can buy for that kind of money.

Of course, if you breed your mare and raise a foal you won't have to pay all that out in a lump sum, but rest assured that your foal will cost that much, a little at a time. Moreover, you never know for sure what kind of a foal your mare will drop. It could be a weakling or a misfit. If you simply buy a colt, you can see what you're getting.

2/ Is my mare worth breeding? If you're planning to breed the mare, you obviously think a lot of her, so answering this question requires real honesty. What outstanding qualities of conformation, color, speed, agility, intelligence, gait, or disposition does she have that you would wish to have transmitted to her offspring? If she has no outstanding qualities, is it really worth the expense of having her produce a foal when it is so much less expensive to simply buy one from a commercial breeder?

3/ Have I selected the proper stallion? Assuming that you have carefully considered the first two questions, and still want to breed your mare, you must now find a stallion. Remember that the foal can't be expected to be any better than its dam and sire. You must therefore pick the best sire possible.

Search the horse magazines for advertisements, and see several studs before making a choice. Never make the mistake of breeding to a horse simply because he is registered and located close to you. No matter how good he is, he may not be right for your mare.

No stallion is perfect. Select one whose qualities will compensate for the weaknesses in your mare. For example, if she's fine-boned and light, look for a stallion with extra muscle in order to get that middle-of-the-road colt you desire. Or, if your mare has a poor head, be sure the stud has a good one and is prepotent enough to put good heads on most of his foals.

Don't select a sire on the basis of cost alone. Don't select a poor stud because the stud fee is $100 less than the good one down the road. Always breed to the very best stallion you can possibly afford. Remember what that foal is going to cost to raise to maturity. What you'll have then depends greatly upon what kind of a horse his sire was. There are too many poor horses around now. We all want to see more good horses. This requires good breeding to start with.

If your mare is worth breeding at all, then she's worth breeding to a good stallion. I don't mean to insinuate that the higher the stud fee, the better the horse. This isn't necessarily so because all good horsemen know high-priced studs that would have been better off gelded and—conversely—some studs with a low stud fee that are truly outstanding. After all, the owner sets the stud fee, not the horse. Generally speaking, of course, one gets what one pays for. If you're an amateur, get the advice of a professional horseman.

Breeding on the Foaling Heat

One of the dilemmas facing the breeder is whether to breed the mare on the foaling heat, or to wait for the second heat.

The advantages of breeding on the foaling heat, which usually starts on the ninth day after foaling, and which is therefore often called the "ninth-day heat," are as follows:

1/ An earlier conception will mean an earlier foal next year, something most breeders desire because it gives the foal an advantage in the show or sales ring, or at the track.

2/ The foaling heat is usually a good strong heat, with the mare very receptive to the stallion and with a good, well-developed ovarian follicle.

The disadvantages of the foaling heat breeding are:

1/ The uterus has not yet involuted (contracted) from the foaling.

2/ The lining of the uterus has not returned to normal. There may be some areas of hemorrhage. Injuries have not had time to heal. The inflamed tissues are more susceptible to infection.

3/ Because of the above factors, the abortion rate on foaling heat conceptions is slightly higher than it is when the mare is bred at a later heat. This fetal loss is *not* high, but it is higher than in mares bred later.

The advantages of breeding at the second or "30-day heat" are:

1/ The uterus is now well involuted, and the uterine tissues more normalized.

2/ Mare and foal are past the stress of the foaling. The foal is stronger and is past the "nine-day scours" (a diarrhea that often occurs in foals when the mare is in the foaling heat).

The disadvantages of breeding at the second heat are:

1/ The conception occurs later and the foal will therefore be born later, and each year the foaling will be at a later date.

2/ Many mares, after having a good foaling heat, with a good follicle, do not have a good subsequent heat. Some suffer lactation anestrus. That is, they don't show another heat while nursing, a serious and frustrating problem for the breeder. Often the follicles are not as good as the foaling heat follicle.

As one reviews the pros and cons of breeding on the foaling heat, one can readily see why the decision is a dilemma for the breeder.

There is, however, a compromise method that, in our practice, has been extremely satisfactory, and that is *not* to breed on the foaling heat, but to recycle the mare prematurely by injecting her with the hormone called prostaglandin. The method is as follows:

1/ Tease the mare daily, noting when the foaling heat begins, and when it ends.

2/ Four or five days after the foaling heat ends, inject the mare with prostaglandin. The timing is important.

3/ Most mares will come back into heat within two to four days after the injection. They usually have a nice big follicle, and they will usually stand for the stallion.

I am ordinarily very conservative about the use of hormones in breeding mares. However, after using this method for several years in our practice I am quite enthusiastic about it. There is only one disadvantage—it is necessary to inject the mare.

There are, on the other hand, many advantages:

1/ We don't have to wait for the 30-day heat. We get an early conception.

2/ The uterus has a few extra days to normalize, and the foal a few extra days to mature before the mare is bred.

3/ We usually get a second heat with a *good* follicle, and the mare is in a strong heat.

In other words, this method gives us the advantages of foal-heat breeding (strong heat, good follicles, and early conception) *plus* the advantages of second-heat breeding (a more normalized uterus and a mare and foal recovered from the stress of foaling).

In our experience, conception rates with this method have been excellent and we have not been able to identify any disadvantages in the method other than the minor trouble and expense involved in administering the hormone to the mare.

Infertility

Every experienced horse breeder will agree that infertility is a major problem. Although modern technology has greatly diminished the number, there are still many mares bred every year that fail to conceive. There are a number of reasons for infertility in mares.

Season: Nature intends for mares to be bred in late spring and early summer.

The foals are then born a year later, when the weather is warm and the feed most abundant and nutritious. Accordingly, mares usually cycle best around the month of May in the Northern Hemisphere, and that is also the time that sperm counts are at their highest in the stallions. But, horse breeders nearly always want early foals. Larger and more mature foals are an advantage in the show ring, the sale barn, or at the track.

The mare's reproductive cycle goes dormant in late summer and remains so through the winter. In late winter, or early spring, the cycle starts again, characterized usually by irregular periods of long heat. This is not the best time to breed mares, but it is the time when most mares are bred. Many, understandably, fail to conceive, and their reproductive cycle may even be disturbed.

The true breeding season, dictated by nature, arriving some months later, is determined by the influence of the increased light of the lengthening daylight hours upon the endocrine glands. More mares would conceive if we waited until nature was ready. However, breeding farms may expose mares to a carefully regulated routine of artificial light, and this technique will encourage most mares to cycle earlier in the year. Consult a veterinarian experienced in broodmare care for an artificial light program suitable for your area.

Grazing spring pastures also seems to ready the mare for breeding. In February, even though mares may show heat periods, the influences of sunlight and green feed are lacking, and, unless artificially compensated for, many mares will fail to settle.

Age: Another factor contributing to infertility is age. When cattle begin to age, they are usually sold for slaughter, not because they are infertile, but because they no longer produce efficiently. By contrast, mares are bred during old age. A good mare is still valuable for breeding even though she can no longer perform physically. Since a certain amount of infertility is to be expected with advancing age, this practice tends to lower the percentage of fertile mares.

One valuable diagnostic technique is the uterine biopsy. It is very easy for a veterinarian, using a special uterine biopsy instrument, to take a snip of tissue from the lining of the mare's uterus. When this is sent to a pathologist trained in the interpretation of such tissue specimens, a quite accurate evaluation can be made of the mare's reproductive potential.

The uterus is then graded, and the diagnosis may range from absolutely hopeless to completely normal. When abnormalities are found, specific treatment can be prescribed that may eliminate some of those abnormalities, actually improving the mare's biopsy rating. Uterine biopsies can be taken on any mare, but they are particularly valuable on the older "problem mare."

Poor Husbandry: Many mares are not properly maintained. Their quarters are cramped. They do not get enough exercise. Faulty nutrition, worminess, and defective teeth are common. These factors contribute to infertility. Excessively fat mares are often hard to settle.

Inheritance: Breeders of horses often have a disregard for fertility, especially in mares. There is a great emphasis upon speed and conformation that yields speed, or emphasis on gaits, athletic prowess, or color. None of these traits contribute to fertility. In fact, there is some evidence that great athletic ability in a mare may actually be conducive to poor reproductive performance. Many fast, powerful mares are hard to settle, and they may be poor milk producers. Yet, such mares are valued as the most desirable broodmares, in the hope that they will transmit their ability to their progeny. It is not surprising that their tendency towards infertility is likewise perpetuated and thus we have many fine racing and performance mares that settle only with great difficulty, often depending upon veterinary intervention.

Poor Breeding Techniques: Some stud farms operate inefficiently and ignorantly. No teasing is done, or it is done improperly. Regular teasing of broodmares by experienced and reliable personnel is absolutely essential for a successful breeding program. There is no substitute for this procedure. The farm must have a good teasing stallion, and the mare handler must be knowledgeable.

Veterinarians can determine if a mare is pregnant, using ultrasonography, after the 15th day, with extreme accuracy. The ultrasound machine can also detect twin pregnancies early. These machines are very expensive, and not all veterinarians or all farms will have ultrasonography available. But an experienced veterinarian can diagnose pregnancy by rectal palpation of the mare's uterus by the 30th day with great accuracy, or even less in many cases.

Yet, many farms do not avail themselves of this service. They simply rebreed the mare if she comes in heat again. This practice is bad because a high percentage of mares will show one or more heats after they conceive. Conversely, some mares that fail to conceive may *not* show a heat subsequently. Thus it becomes impossible to determine if a mare is failing to conceive, or is conceiving and then losing and resorbing the embroyo early in pregnancy.

Early pregnancy diagnosis is an essential and integral part of every scientific breeding program. An increasingly popular diagnostic tool is uterine endoscopy, also known as hysteroscopy. This is a technique involving examination of the interior of the uterus with a fiberoptic endoscope. Some practices are even using video endoscopy. A film is made of the examination. This is rather expensive.

Incidentally, in my experience, blood testing is an inferior and less reliable method of diagnosing pregnancy than either ultrasound or rectal palpation, both of which are extremely accurate. Blood testing also fails to offer a variety of other information that the veterinarian gains by actually palpating the uterus and the ovaries of the mare.

Sanitation and skill in handling mares is also lacking on some farms.

Infection: Infection of the reproductive tract is said to be the single greatest cause of infertility. This may be true, but the breeder cannot fail to consider the causes we have already mentioned. I personally believe that too much emphasis has been placed on infection. We must remember that the external genitalia of all mares have microorganisms living therein, and that this is entirely normal. However, true infection can and does occur, and it will certainly interfere with fertility.

No well-managed stud farm will

accept a mare unless she is accompanied by a certificate signed by a veterinarian certifying her to have normal genitalia, and that she is free of infection. When we do such a pre-breeding exam, it includes examination of the vulva, the vagina, the cervix, preferably when the mare is in heat. A bacteriological culture is then taken from inside the uterus. A rectal examination is performed, so the uterus and the ovaries can be palpated. The presence of follicles is noted.

If the culture yields a significant bacterial growth, tests are run to determine which antibiotics the organism is sensitive to, so appropriate treatment can be prescribed.

Anatomy: Many infections in mares are caused indirectly by anatomical peculiarities. Some of these may be obvious, even to the layman, but others can only be detected by internal examination. We are discussing such problems as distortion of the vulva (usually from lacerations incurred at foaling time), tilting of the vulva (exposing the vagina to contamination with manure), tilting of the vagina (causing "pooling" of urine within the vagina), and distortions of the cervix (from foaling injury or from breeding injury).

But, not all infections in mares are due to anatomical faults. Some are transmitted venereally. Many are due to dirty breeding techniques. Some just happen. And, I believe that many are introduced when breeding mares at the foaling heat (the first heat after foaling, usually around the ninth day).

There are other anatomical causes of infertility. These include closed tubes, hermaphroditism, imperforate hymen, and various other congenital or accidental problems.

Endocrine Imbalance: To the owner of the mare, the first thought that often occurs when a mare fails to settle is, "Have the vet give her a hormone shot." Ah, if only it were that simple.

Hormone imbalances do occur in horses, and they are by no means rare. But, as in infection, don't disregard all the other factors we have cited that contribute to sterility. Diagnosing endocrine abnormalities is difficult. Some are detected readily, others only after repeated pelvic examinations every day or two, and some only by blood testing to assay hormone levels.

Some of these conditions will respond to treatment with hormones and some will not. Do not expect the veterinarian to glance at a mare that has failed to settle, give her a magical hormone shot, and solve the problem. It is a much more complicated business than that.

In recent years, great strides have been made in our ability to control the cycle of mares using hormones. With progesterones we can regulate the cycle, and these hormones can now be given by mouth. The prostaglandins have been invaluable for a variety of purposes, but particularly to recycle mares more quickly and control the timing of follicle formation. Other hormones, like estrogens and follicle-stimulating hormones and chorionic gonadotrophin, are all very useful.

Miscellaneous Causes of Infertility: Sometimes we see an infertile mare to which none of the above-mentioned causes can apply. She is physically normal. She cycles regularly. But she fails to conceive. There are mares that have a reaction to the stallion's semen and actually reject it. There are problems we cannot identify and do not yet understand. In some cases there are psychological reasons for sterility. The emotions and the endocrine system are closely linked. If a sensitive mare is hauled in a trailer, unloaded in a strange place, surrounded by strangers, restrained with a twitch and with breeding hobbles, and exposed to a stallion she doesn't know, isn't it logical that the psychological shock might interfere with a successful breeding? I think so.

The Stallion: We have listed nine reasons the mare may fail to conceive, but we haven't mentioned one other: the infertile stallion. The totally sterile stallion is obvious. He will sire no foals. The real problem is the stallion with impaired fertility. He settles some mares but not others, and the mares get the blame. He can be detected by a laboratory examination of a semen sample. Remember that semen quality can vary. It may be poor if a stallion hasn't been bred for a long time. Conversely, if a stallion is being used heavily, the sperm count may also be temporarily lowered. If semen of poor quality is found, it is important, therefore, to collect and examine additional specimens. Wise stallion owners will periodically have their stallions checked. If it serves no other purpose, the unhappy owner of a barren mare can be assured that the problem lies with the mare, and not with the stallion.

Follicle Palpation: The ovaries of the mare can be felt through the rectum. The growing follicle can be identified, and we can tell when rupture of the follicle, with release of the egg, is imminent. That's the time to breed the mare, even if the mare disagrees. Breeding "on the follicle" is, to me, the single most important thing (along with proper teasing by the farm) that has enabled veterinarians to help settle "problem mares."

Add to that uterine cultures, uterine endoscopy, cycle control with oral progesterone and prostaglandins, surgery to correct anatomic defects, rhinopneumonitis vaccine, and hormones to prevent abortion, and techniques such as artificial insemination and embryo transfer, and we have the tools to completely maximize foaling percentages.

Foaling

If your mare is in foal, now is the time to review the duties of equine midwifery—before the foal arrives. Mares seldom have obstetrical difficulties—much less often than cattle, for example—but when a mare does have trouble, the situation is a grave emergency.

The muscles of the mare are very powerful, and if she is in trouble, the foal will not survive long and, in fact, the loss of the mare as well is quite likely. To use cattle again as a comparison, the cow experiencing a complicated labor can survive many hours, even days.

Pregnancy in the mare lasts about 11 months. However, normal foals may be delivered in the tenth month, or as late as 12½ months. So do not panic if your mare goes past the 11-month date. If it is her first foal, she is especially likely to run close to 12 months. The majority of mares will deliver between 340 and 350 days after conceiving.

Difficulties are less likely to occur at foaling time if the mare is not too fat and has been properly fed and exercised throughout the pregnancy. We recommend the mare be ridden daily, or otherwise exercised, right up to the day she foals. Care should be taken, however, not to exhaust her, or allow her to become winded or overheated.

Mares usually foal at night. No matter how hard they try, inexperienced owners will rarely be able to detect the signs of imminent labor in the mare. Frequently, the owner stays up many nights to attend the foaling, and finally gives up the project in discouragement. Then, one morning, there is the new foal.

As I said, mares rarely get into trouble, so statistically the odds are that all will be well whether the foaling is supervised or not. In fact, a nervous novice can do more harm than good. But, because a mare in trouble constitutes a serious emergency, the foaling should be observed whenever possible.

As the foaling date approaches, the mare should ideally be provided a roomy, clean, dry, well-bedded foaling stall. It is a good idea to bandage her tail and wash her hindquarters with warm, soapy water before delivery. Don't forget to remove the bandage after the foaling.

Experienced horsemen can usually detect the signs of parturition. The tissues around the base of the tail seem to sink. The udder is swollen, and a waxlike discharge forms on the ends of the teats in most cases.

The first sign of labor is restlessness. The mare may act colicky and paw the ground. The first contractions are gentle. The birth canal dilates. Soon the water bag protrudes from the vulva. *Do not* break it.

Most mares will lie down at this point. The contractions grow stronger. Normally, both forelegs are presented. *Do not* pull on the legs. Two or three contractions later, and the head of the foal appears. The mare will usually look around at this point. Then, with surprising swiftness and a few final expulsive efforts, the foal will be delivered rather suddenly.

If all goes as we have described, do not interfere or attempt to assist. Stay out of the stall. If, however, you see any deviation from the process described, phone your veterinarian. Active labor in the mare should only last 15 or 20 minutes. If it lasts more than half an hour, there is a great likelihood of losing the

Mares usually foal at night. No matter how hard they try, inexperienced owners will rarely be able to detect the signs of imminent labor in the mare.

133

foal. If you see only one foot presented, or a head and no feet, or two feet and no head, or soles of feet pointing upward instead of downward, phone for help. If the foal's muzzle is still in the sack, or covered with mucus or membranes, the muzzle should be exposed so the foal can breathe.

Shortly after the foal is born the mare will get up. As she does so, the umbilical cord will break. It is connected to the afterbirth, which usually is still inside the mare. Once in a while the afterbirth comes out with the foal. In such cases, you may have to free the foal from the membranes, but this does not happen often.

Remember, allow the mare to stand when she is ready. Do not rush her. Do not cut the cord. Allow it to break naturally. This is to ensure that all of the blood in the afterbirth has a chance to enter the foal.

The mare will usually lick the foal. Mares do not eat the afterbirth. It should fall from the mare within a half hour or so. If the afterbirth is retained for a few hours, better inform your veterinarian so that he can make plans to remove it. A retained placenta can result in lamini-

tis (founder). If the afterbirth comes out of its own accord, save it, because your veterinarian may want to examine it later.

Some high-strung young mares panic when they get up and discover the afterbirth hanging from them. They may go into a kicking frenzy. Such mares should be haltered before they arise, and a competent horseman should restrain them until they settle down.

Many mares are very jealous about their foals, and they can become aggressive. Ordinarily gentle mares might become quite vicious after foaling, so be careful.

After the cord breaks off the foal, the stump should be disinfected by immersion in disinfectant. A small, wide-mouthed bottle is ideal. Keep the foal dry and warm. It is all right to rub it down with clean, dry towels. When the foal feels strong enough, it will struggle to its feet and start hunting for the mare's udder. Don't panic if the newborn foal's legs look weak or crooked. Most of them do. If the mare will not allow the foal to nurse, tie up one front leg long enough for a nursing. In some cases, the mare will require a twitch or tranquilizer.

If the foal's muzzle is still in the sack, or covered with mucus or membranes, the muzzle should be exposed so the foal can breathe.

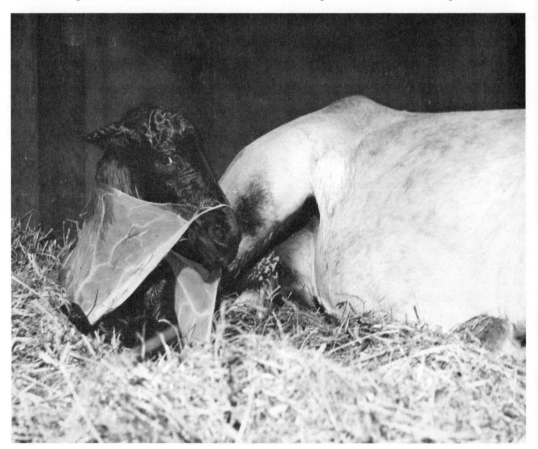

Most veterinarians like to see the mare and foal within the first 24 hours. Both will be examined for abnormalities. Inoculations and protective injections will usually be given. We always give the foal an enema to help empty the meconium (fetal stool) from its rectum, because foals are more prone to serious constipation than other newborn animals.

This is also the time for the veterinarian to inspect the afterbirth to be sure it has been completely delivered, and to check the premises and fences to see if the environment is safe for the foal. The future care and feeding of mare and foal can be discussed at this time, too.

Raising the Orphan Foal

Caring for an orphan foal is hard work, especially during the first week of its life, but those who have done it successfully will agree that it is a satisfying experience. There is many a fine horse at whom the owner points a prideful finger saying, "I raised him on a bottle."

A foal may be orphaned in several ways. Often a mare will refuse to accept her foal. Such a mare should be tranquilized. If she continues to reject her foal it may be necessary to restrain her with a twitch. I've had good luck tying up one front leg on such mares, in order to give the foal a chance to nurse. A foal may also be orphaned because the mare cannot produce any milk. Lastly, a foal is sometimes literally orphaned by the loss or death of its dam.

Whatever the reason, the person bearing the responsibility of caring for such a foal has undertaken a real job.

The first milk, or colostrum, is important for any newborn animal. It is very rich and has a high vitamin content. It is filled with disease-fighting antibodies. Colostrum also has a laxative action, thereby helping to clear the foal's bowel of meconium (fetal intestinal contents). Nature provides colostrum, with its special protective properties, to aid the newborn during the first critical days of life. It is a good idea for breeding farms to keep some colostrum in the freezer.

The foal that is deprived of colostrum is more susceptible to infection, constipation, and other serious afflictions of the newborn. To compensate for this lack, veterinarians usually prescribe high levels of antibiotics for such foals, plus supplemental vitamins by mouth or injection, and enemas to prevent death

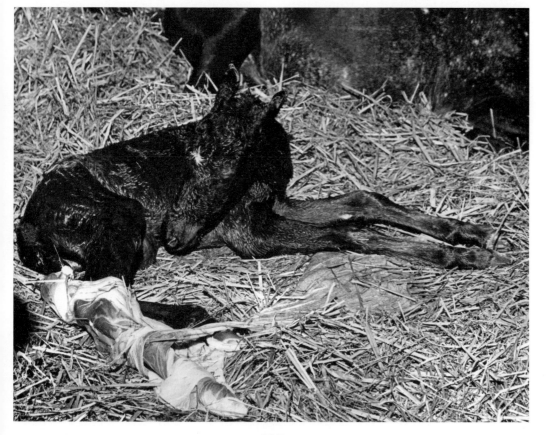

Remember, allow the mare to stand when she is ready. Do not rush her. Do not cut the cord. Allow it to break naturally.

due to severe constipation. Protective serum may also be given and commercial plasma is now available.

Naturally, the foal will also need protection from extreme temperatures and dampness. Excessive warmth is not recommended if the foal is alert and active.

The other thing our orphan will need is food, and this is the most time-consuming part of the job. The baby foal should be fed every hour, taking about half a pint, more or less, depending upon the size of the foal. After a couple of days the interval between feedings may be increased to two hours, and in a week or so to four hours. Don't expect the foal to do well unless you are willing to feed it *frequently*. By one month of age, four feedings a day will do. The commonest question the owner asks is "What do I feed this foal?"

If mare's milk is available, naturally it is best. Sometimes a nurse mare is available, or a mare may be milked and the foal bottle-fed. Most foals will nurse from a bottle fitted with a large calf or lamb nipple. Weak foals may be fed by having a veterinarian pass a tube through a nostril, down to the stomach. If necessary such a nasogastric tube may be left in place temporarily. Most foals will soon learn to drink milk from a pan, and eventually from a bucket.

But usually mare's milk isn't available, and a substitute formula must be used. Mare's milk is lower in protein, and the protein is different than cow's milk. It is also lower in fat, but is higher in sugar. Therefore, we can modify cow's milk to approximate mare's milk by lowering the protein and fat content, modifying the nature of the protein, and increasing the sugar content.

There are many formulas that accomplish this. In fact, a check of 16 sources (4 universities, 6 textbooks, and 6 veterinarians) yielded 16 formulas. Though they all varied, their objective was as described above, and remember that the milk of mares will vary considerably from one animal to another. Any of the following formulas may be tried. If one doesn't agree with the foal, try another.

FORMULA No. 1
1 pint of low-fat cow's milk
4 ounces of lime water
1 teaspoon of sugar

FORMULA No. 2
1 pint of low-fat cow's milk
2½ ounces of water
2½ ounces of lime water
2 teaspoons of lactose

FORMULA No. 3
1 can evaporated cow's milk
1 can of water
4 tablespoons of lime water
1 tablespoon of sugar or corn syrup

By low-fat milk, we do not mean non-fat (skim) milk, but cow's milk with a butterfat content of 1 percent to 2 percent. Regular cow's milk has a butterfat content of 2½ to 7 percent depending upon the cow. Market whole milk is usually standardized to 2½ to 3½ percent. In many areas, the markets carry low-fat milk, so labelled.

Goat's milk has been used successfully, although its formula really is not too close to mare's milk, In fact, foals can be taught to suck a good nanny.

Commercial mare's milk substitutes are available, such as Foal-Lac, and they work well if the instructions are followed.

Regardless of the formula used, bring it to body temperature (about 100 degrees Fahrenheit) before feeding. If the foal will not eat, or shows signs of weakness, illness, fever, diarrhea, or constipation, call your veterinarian at once. Modern drugs, intravenous feedings, plasma and transfusions can save many foals nowadays that used to die, but it is important to initiate treatment before they are too far gone.

As soon as the foal is interested, allow it free access to green grass, or top quality leafy alfalfa hay. When the foal will eat grain, see that a mixture is available. There are many good formulas. Here is a simple one:
1/ Steamed rolled oats, 80 percent
2/ Linseed meal, 10 percent
3/ Wheat bran, 10 percent
Half the oats may be replaced with barley if desired. Offer a hundred-pound foal a half-pound of this grain ration daily. Increase the grain proportionately as the foal grows. Add a balanced vitamin-mineral supplement as directed on the label. Many feed suppliers now manufacture pelleted formulas, specially designed for young foals. Many such

products are advertised in your horse magazines.

Parasite control and vaccinations are important for any foal, but this is especially true for the orphan foal because he is at a nutritional disadvantage.

Newborn foals shouldn't be left alone. Leave them with a friendly goat, duck, burro, dog, cat, or other animal for company.

Umbilical Diseases of Foals

The umbilical cord, or navel cord as it is also called, is the cord that connects the unborn foal to the placental sacs that surround it. The cord serves to nourish the developing foal, and also to carry away waste products. Blood vessels in it carry blood from the placenta to the foal, and back again. The cord also contains a tube called the urachus that connects to the foal's bladder, and carries off urinary waste to the outer water bag.

The umbilical cord is an important organ, for without it the foal could not grow and survive inside the uterus of the mare. When the foal is born, the cord breaks and seals itself off. The foal is thereafter on its own and must depend upon nursing for its source of food, breathing for its air supply, and must urinate and pass manure in order to rid its body of waste material. The stump of the cord shrivels and dries up, and eventually falls away, leaving the scar we know as the umbilicus, or navel, or "belly button."

When a foal is born, the owner may be tempted to tie off and cut the umbilical cord. Don't do this. You may deprive the foal of a large amount of blood which is in the placenta (afterbirth) and thereby weaken the foal. Don't hurry the delivery. The foal will be delivered before the placenta. You will notice that the foal is attached by the thick umbilical cord to the placenta, which usually remains in the mare for quite a while. The blood in the placenta will drain into the foal and, as the mare stands, the umbilical cord will rupture, bleed for a little while, and then contract.

As soon after this as possible, dip the end of the cord into a bottle of whatever disinfectant your veterinarian prefers.

Ordinarily, no other treatment is necessary. If you wish, the stump of the cord may be dusted with a medicated powder to help dry it up.

If it is absolutely necessary to cut the cord artificially, disinfect it with iodine, tie it off with two sterile ligatures, and cut between them. The cord normally has an indented breaking point about two inches from the body. This is the place to cut it.

This organ, in foals, more than any other species of animal, is prone to several disease conditions. These include: umbilical hernia, pervious urachus, and navel ill. Let's discuss these one at a time.

Umbilical hernia or omphalocele is very common in foals. It is, in fact, the most frequent hernia seen in horses, or in any other domestic animal. In an umbilical hernia there is an opening in the belly muscles due to a weakening at the navel. Some intestine, or membrane inside the belly, protrudes through this opening, covered with skin, of course. The result is a bulge at the navel of the foal, the size of a golf ball, or larger. If you feel the bulge, you can detect the contents inside of it, and also usually push a finger up through the opening into the abdominal cavity. The hernia occurs at birth, or shortly after, and is considered to be a birth defect. Some hernias may be due to straining such as occurs when a foal has diarrhea or constipation, or from constant nickering when separated from its dam.

Many umbilical hernias disappear without treatment by the time the foal is a yearling. If not, surgery will be required. If you detect a hernia in a foal, it should be examined by a veterinarian. He will decide whether it should be left alone and given a chance to disappear by itself. Or, he may decide that it is a larger hernia, in danger of strangulating, and recommend surgery.

It used to be popular to apply blisters to umbilical hernias, or inject irritants into them to try to scar them closed. Such methods usually fail, and the resulting scar tissue may make subsequent surgery more difficult. Surgical correction of a hernia may be "open" or "closed." In the closed method, the hernia is clamped off with special clamps or ligatures. Great skill is necessary to do this properly. In the open method, the

Some hernias may be due to straining such as occurs when a foal has diarrhea or constipation, or from constant nickering when separated from its dam.

hernia is closed by one of several operations. The veterinarian will select the technique he feels is best capable of handling the particular hernia.

Pervious or open urachus is seen much less often. In the opening paragraph we described the function of the urachus. We mentioned that along with the umbilical blood vessels, the urachus closes after birth. However, once in a while it remains open, and urine will then drip from the umbilical cord especially when the foal is urinating. The stump of the cord is therefore always wet. An open urachus is serious and your veterinarian should close it, surgically, if necessary, to prevent infection. It is not, however, an emergency.

Navel ill, or *omphalophlebitis*, is one of the most serious diseases in foals. After the cord ruptures, germs can easily enter the open end, causing infection. This infection may then spread to the liver. Or, it may spread by way of the urachus into the urinary system, and from there into the entire bloodstream causing septicemia. This may quickly kill the foal, or the infection may spread elsewhere in the body, especially into the joints, causing "joint ill," wherein the joints fill with pus. Many foals have been so ruined.

Naturally, navel ill occurs most often in foals born in dirty barns and corrals. You can help prevent navel ill in several ways. Don't forget to dip the stump of the cord in a disinfectant. Let it soak a bit. Provide a clean place for the mare to foal, such as an open pasture or a stall with plenty of fresh bedding. Your veterinarian may decide to give the foal antitoxin or antibiotics after foaling, to help avoid navel infections.

Diseases of Foals

Most baby foals are vigorous, self-sufficient individuals. Happily, they are not particularly prone to troubles as compared with some other animals. However, difficulties inevitably occur, and the breeder must familiarize himself with these difficulties and learn how to prevent them, or cope with them if they happen in spite of precautions.

Let's investigate some baby foal diseases.

Hemolytic disease: This serious disease is known by many names such as *Neonatal isoerythrolysis, hemolytic disease, icteric foals, jaundiced foals, Rh factor, Hemolytic icterus, Hemolytic anemic,* and *Icterus gravis.* Some of these names are more appropriate than others. Technically, *Neonatal isoerythrolysis* is the most acceptable at this time. In this disease, an allergic reaction occurs between the red blood cells of the foal and antibodies found in the colostrum or first milk of the mare. When the newborn foal nurses, the antibodies are swallowed and absorbed. They attack the foal's red blood cells and destroy them, causing anemia. The hemoglobin pigments released from the destroyed cells are picked up by the tissues, causing yellow jaundice (or icterus). This condition is usually seen in mares that have had three or four foals. It is rare in mares in foal for the first time.

Icteric foals occur in all breeds, but by far are most often seen in the Thoroughbred and also in mule foals. The anemic foal shows weakness even before he is obviously jaundiced. He must be immediately removed from his dam and a veterinarian called. Tests run upon the sire's or foal's blood and the mare's serum or colostrum will confirm the diagnosis. This disease is similar to Rh disease of human babies. Most untreated cases die before they are four days old. Very acute cases may die the first day, in which case jaundice does not have time to develop. Usually the affected foal, in addition to yellow jaundice, shows lethargy, rapid pulse and respirations, and sometimes discolored urine.

Many icteric foals can be saved if removed from the mare soon enough and put on a formula instead. Meanwhile the mare is milked out hourly to eliminate all the antibody-containing colostrum. The foal frequently will require blood transfusions in order to have a chance of survival. Blood tests tell the veterinarian whether the foal needs blood, and how much it will require.

Breeders should learn how to prevent foal losses from this disease. The mare's blood serum may be tested against the sire's blood cells a week or two prior to the expected foaling date. A positive reaction means that the foal must not be allowed to nurse the mare until it is three days old. After the second day, the foal can no longer absorb the lethal antibodies. Meanwhile the mare may be milked out. The foal is best muzzled to prevent nursing.

Once a mare has produced an icteric foal, special precautions should be taken to protect future foals. Ideally, she should be bred to a stallion with a compatible blood type. This is determined by blood tests. The foal produced by this breeding will be safe.

If she *must* be bred to a stallion with incompatible blood, the foal might be saved by observing the following precautions: be present when the foal is born and muzzle it immediately upon delivery; have your veterinarian run tests upon the foal's blood and the mare's colostrum to see if the milk is safe. If it is not safe, the foal must be fed colostrum from a different mare while the dam is milked out hourly until tests show that the milk is safe, or until the foal is three days old.

Actinobacillosis: Actinobacillosis used to be called *Viscosum infection* or *shigellosis.* It is a very serious bacterial infection of baby foals, and sometimes older horses. Affected foals are often called "sleepers" or "dummy foals" by breeders. The symptoms in baby foals include diarrhea, swollen joints, general illness, weakness, refusal to nurse, and high fever. "Sleeper" foals simply lie in a semiconscious state, making occasional weak leg movements. Dummy foals wander about stupidly, in an incoordinate manner. Sleeper and dummy foals are sometimes the result of other infections besides actinobacillosis.

Many of these foals may be saved if the veterinarian will help to prevent actinobacillosis. Wrap the mare's tail and wash her hindquarters prior to foaling. Wash the udder too. Disinfect the foal's navel with iodine or Betadine. Provide clean bedding.

In Europe, a convulsive syndrome of newborn Thoroughbred foals is seen. These foals are also called dummy foals (or wanderers or barkers). The cause of this syndrome is not definitely known, but it is *not* due to actinobacillosis. Many of these foals recover with no treatment except forced feeding. Foals suffering from actinobacillosis in the United States will not survive this minimal treatment. I mention this lest someone be led astray by advice regarding dummy foals in a European book.

Diarrhea: Diarrhea in the baby foal is often due to intestinal upset caused by greedy nursing when the mare is a heavy milker, eating excessive manure (most foals will eat some manure, which is probably nature's way of establishing microorganisms in the digestive tract), or at the ninth day or shortly thereafter from the mare coming into heat. But diarrhea may also be the first sign of actinobacillosis or other fatal infections. *Never* neglect diarrhea in a foal. It should be carefully examined, the cause of the diarrhea determined, and appropriate measures taken to stop it at once. All baby animals are weakened and dehydrated very quickly by diarrhea, and their body defenses markedly lowered.

Constipation: Young foals are uniquely predisposed to constipation, and neglected cases frequently die from bowel obstruction. The foal is born with stool in his large intestine. This fetal stool is called *meconium.* It is firm and dark in color. The foal should have bowel movements regularly, from the time it is foaled. Colostrum is very laxative, and is nature's way of cleaning out the meconium. I personally believe that every newborn foal should have an enema as part of the routine post-partum care.

Constipated foals will strain to defecate, switch their tails, and stamp their feet. They must be promptly relieved or the colon will gradually plug up for a distance of two or three feet, causing a potentially fatal obstruction.

Contracted tendons and crooked feet: Many foals are born with weak legs, crooked feet, or contracted tendons. Some cases will straighten up without treatment. In other cases the veterinarian may have to resort to braces, casts, or orthopedic surgery to save the foal.

Besides the common conditions mentioned above, foals may have many congenital defects, or they may acquire many diseases and problems during the first week or two of life. Foaling problems are minimized by seeing that the pregnant mare is well-nourished, free of worms, and exercised. Whenever possible the foaling should be attended by an experienced person, and a veterinarian called the moment any difficulty occurs.

Every foal should be examined by a competent veterinarian soon after delivery, and routine post-partum care administered. A newborn foal is usually the result of a costly breeding and a year of pregnancy. If it dies, all that is wasted, and more than another year will go by before the mare can deliver another. Two years is a long time. There are, therefore, no "'cheap" foals, and no expense should be spared to ensure the survival of a foal.

Sometimes we run special tests. For example, if the foal is an Arabian, a CID test may be desired to check for Combined Immuno-Deficiency, an inheritable blood disorder seen in some Arabian foals. The immune systems of foals with CID cannot produce antibodies, and after several months these foals usually die.

In foals of any breed an FPT test can be run; FPT stands for Failure of Passive Transfer. This blood test, run eight or more hours after the foal has first nursed, tells us whether the foal has picked up protective antibodies from the colostrum to protect him against infection. There are a number of reasons a foal may have failed to receive passive antibodies from the colostrum, even though he has nursed. First of all, the mare may have inadequate antibodies herself, thereby having colostrum that is inadequate.

Secondly, the mare's colostrum may have been normal, but she may have lost it all. This often occurs in mares that leak or squirt milk before the foal is born. You see, the protective antibodies are only in the very first milk—the colostrum. If the colostrum all leaks out, only ordinary milk is left by the time the foal is born. That foal will not be adequately protected against infection. That's why some seemingly vigorous foals soon come down with a bowel infection, or pneumonia, or septicemia, and die despite treatment.

Lastly, the colostrum may be normal, but the foal may simply be unable to pick up the antibodies in it, and that foal, again, will be unprotected. If the FPT test indicates an inadequate level of protective antibodies, the foal can be protected with injections of plasma, and perhaps with antibiotics. If an FPT test is desired, ask your veterinarian to run one when you make your appointment. FPT is not common, but foals do die every year from it. The test is not terribly expensive and it can prevent a needless tragedy.

At the time of birth, it is wise to protect the foal against tetanus with antitoxin. Don't confuse this with tetanus toxoid. Antitoxin gives the immediate but temporary protection against tetanus, but it is *not* a vaccination, and the foal will have to be immunized when he is a little older. Newborn foals *can* get tetanus, probably through the navel, and I have seen a few such cases. It also helps to booster the mare's immunity late in pregnancy, thereby ensuring a maximum level of antibodies in the colostrum, or first milk.

I like to check the premises to be sure they are safe for the foal, but ideally this should be done long before the foal is born.

In my own practice, losses of newborn foals are much lower when thorough post-partum care is given than it is in the uncared-for foals. For example, joint ill used to be very common in our practice, crippling or killing many foals. Today, it is a rare disease, probably because of good post-partum care.

Once the foal is past the first few critical weeks, don't relax your vigilance. Keep him wormed, be sure your fences are safe, creep feed him, vaccinate him, give him room to exercise, halter break and gentle him, and keep his feet trimmed. Your reward will be a sleek, glossy, active foal. It is unfair to bring a foal into the world, and then allow him to deteriorate into a wormy, pot-bellied, unthrifty mess.

CPR in the Newborn Foal

Most informed people today are familiar with CPR (cardiopulmonary resuscitation) in the human being. Those who are not should become so, because lives can be saved with CPR. Many victims of heart attack, drowning, and electric shock are alive today because somebody knew how to administer CPR.

It is taught in schools, in industry, by organizations such as the Red Cross, and by many medical facilities. Descriptive placards are displayed in many public places, such as swimming pools.

CPR is used when a person's heart has stopped (called cardiac arrest) or when breathing has stopped (respiratory arrest). When the heart has stopped, some degree of blood circulation can be maintained by applying rhythmic hand pressure to the victim's chest. When breathing has stopped, air can be forced into the lungs of the victim by blowing into his mouth while simultaneously pinching off his nostrils.

If the heart and breathing have both stopped, both cardiac and pulmonary resuscitation must be applied—and often the victim can be kept alive.

Newborn foals sometimes require CPR. Therefore it is important to know how to give CPR to a foal, and to understand that it is done differently than it is in a human.

The most common cause of cardiac and/or respiratory arrest in a newborn foal is prolonged or complicated labor by the mare. Usually the respiratory arrest occurs first. When a foal is deprived of oxygen for too long, cardiac arrest follows.

When the foal is in the mare's uterus, it does not breathe. It gets its oxygen supply from the mare by way of the placenta and the umbilical cord. The heart is working, of course, and has been since the foal was a tiny embryo.

In a normal foaling, which is a swift procedure in mares, the separation of the foal from the mare usually occurs when the umbilical cord ruptures, after the foal has been born. It is best to allow this to occur naturally.

If the cord is cut or tied off prematurely, the foal may be deprived of a significant amount of blood from the placenta, which will ordinarily drain into the foal's body through the umbilical blood vessels. Sometimes the placenta will be delivered with the foal, although in most cases it remains behind, to drop from the mare later. In either case, as soon as the foal loses its oxygen source (the mare), its brain is signalled to commence breathing.

Sometimes the umbilical cord is crushed while the foal's head is still inside the mare; or if the head has come out, it may still be in the water bag. Or perhaps the foal is coming out hind feet first. In such cases, if the umbilical source of oxygen is interrupted, the

The large X marks the spot where cardiac resuscitation is applied to a foal.

Knowing how to apply CPR to a foal whose heart is not beating or who is not breathing might save his life.

foal's brain will be signalled to start breathing. By inhaling fluids, instead of dry outside air, a foal will drown.

Saving it then becomes a matter of CPR.

If the foal is not breathing, feel the chest, behind the elbow. Is there a heartbeat? If there *is* a heartbeat, you do not need to do cardiac massage. Instead, start respiratory resuscitation as follows:

1/ Clear the nose of fluids. These may be sucked out with a syringe, but what I usually do is pick up the foal by the hind end, and whirl it in a circle a few times. Centrifugal force will expel fluids and mucus in the upper respiratory tract. Now, quickly begin the pulmonary resuscitation.

2/ Close off one nostril. Blow into the other nostril. Unlike humans, horses cannot breathe through their mouth, so *do not blow into the mouth.*

By closing off one nostril and blowing into the other, you will effectively fill the lungs with air. A foal's lungs are approximately the same size as a human's, so unless you are dealing with a tiny pony foal or miniature horse foal, you don't have to worry about overinflating the lungs. Just take a deep breath, blow all you can into the foal's nostril while pinching off the other.

You should see the chest expand as the lungs fill with air. Then pause a moment as the lungs collapse and expel the air. Repeat this procedure, rhythmically. The rate is the same as you yourself normally breathe. Just breathe *in* deeply and slowly, and breathe *out* into the foal's nostril.

If the foal starts to cough and sputter, stop for a moment to see if it has begun breathing on its own and, if so, if the breathing is strong and regular.

3/ If the heart has also stopped, then complete CPR is necessary. This can be done by one person, but it isn't easy. You will need to stuff something up one of the foal's nostrils to close it off while you blow in the other as already described. This will free your hands to do cardiac massage. Obviously, it is much better if one person can do the pulmonary resuscitation, while the second person does the following cardiac massage.

4/ With the foal lying on its *right* side, place both hands over the lower left chest wall, just behind the foal's elbow. One hand should be on top of the other. The heel of the lower hand contacts the chest wall where the heart is most superficial.

With sharp but not excessive force, compress the heart and then immediately release the pressure. Repeat at one-second intervals. Violent force can rupture the heart. It only takes a moderate force to compress the heart and pump blood out of it.

In human CPR, the patient lies on his or her back, while similar massage is given to the heart by compressing the chest. In the horse, the chest has a different shape, and therefore the equine patient must lie on its side.

Of course, if you feel the heartbeat start under your hand, and if it is beating regularly, stop the cardiac massage, but watch carefully in case the heart stops again.

If oxygen is available (and serious breeding farms should have an oxygen tank available, equipped with a reducing valve and a length of plastic tubing), then oxygen may be simultaneously given during CPR. To do this, run the plastic tube up the nostril being pinched off, about as far as the distance to the foal's eye. Then go on with the resuscitation.

To Summarize:

Learn CPR for humans. It may save a life and the technique is the same as will be used in a newborn foal except that in the foal, we do not do mouth-to-mouth resuscitation. Instead, we do mouth-to-nostril resuscitation, closing off the opposite nostril by pinching it with our fingers or by stuffing something up the nostril (a tennis ball works perfectly in a full-sized horse, but you'll need something smaller in a foal).

Also, in humans, cardiac massage is performed with the patient lying on his or her back. In foals, the patient must lie on its right side.

Feeding Growing Foals

Conservative and simple feeding programs are recommended for growing foals. Elaborate rations designed to accelerate growth at abnormal rates are often responsible for metabolic and skeletal abnormalities in young horses. Nature designed the horse to nurse while it is young, and to graze grass (including the seeds, which we call grain) for all of its life. Our common sense feeding program is based upon this premise. Keep in mind, however, that this program is a starting point. Foals vary in their needs and this program may be tailored to the individual foal.

Let's define some terms used in this discussion.

Roughage—Pasture, or hay in any form: loose, baled, pelleted, cubed, or chopped.

Milk replacer—Specific mare's-milk substitutes such as Foal-Lac or Start-To-Finish, etc.

Milk supplement—General milk replacers such as Calf Manna and Manomar, etc.

Creep mix—Commercially prepared pelleted ration for creep feeding.

Concentrates—Can be categorized in three areas: 1/ Grain, such as oats or barley or corn; 2/ Grain mixes containing several grains and milling by-products, usually sweetened with molasses; 3/ Pelleted concentrates such as Broodmare and Foal Pellets.

THE SUCKLING FOAL

Following birth, the foal needs only its dam's milk. Soon, it will start to nibble hay and grain. Creep feeding is not mandatory the first couple of months, but mare and foal will usually do better if creep feeding is started earlier. In the creep, the foal should be offered roughage plus a mixture of one-half milk replacer and one-half sweet grain mix. Or, you may feed commercially prepared creep mix along with the roughage if you prefer.

THE WEANLING

Foals may be weaned at *any* age, and raised to healthy maturity. All weanlings need roughage, plus a milk replacer if less than six months of age, and a milk supplement if more than six months of age. In addition, feed one-half pound of grain per 100 pounds of body weight daily, divided into two feedings. In other words, a 400-pound weanling would get one pound of grain twice daily. The grain can be a commercial mix, or you can use rolled oats or barley. Many sources advise much heavier grain allowances than this, but to do so increases the probability of the foal developing epiphysitis and other bone damage, and contracted tendons.

A vitamin-mineral supplement is okay, but use only one product, and follow the instructions on the label.

Weanlings may even be conditioned to show at halter on such a diet. There are pellets under various names that may be fed free choice along with the above grain rations and some milk supplement.

Foals fed in this manner will be fat, yet not have a big hay belly, and not be consuming dangerously high levels of grain.

THE YEARLING

The yearling needs ample roughage, plus one-half pound of concentrate for 100 pounds of body weight daily. As they mature, some yearlings will require a little more concentrate. Others will require less. A milk supplement will help ensure adequate protein and mineral levels, as will a vitamin-mineral supplement.

Weaning

If the nursing mare is not pregnant, and neither mare nor foal are needed for work or show, there is no need to hurry the weaning time. Most mares will wean a foal of their own accord before the foal reaches yearling status. If the owner finds it inconvenient to let the foal nurse this long, then weaning may be started at seven or eight months of age.

If the mare is pregnant and especially if she was bred soon after foaling, then the nursing foal should be weaned at six months of age. A mare in foal and still nursing a foal over six months old is likely to become weakened and anemic by the strain upon her system. If necessary, foals can be weaned much earlier.

Some owners find weaning a major chore, and it really shouldn't be that big of a job. The foal ready to be weaned should already be on a substantial grain and supplement ration, and free of internal parasites. Then simply separate the mare and foal completely. If the foal and dam are out of earshot and cannot see each other, they will quickly adjust to the separation. However, weaning also can be handled in adjacent pens (provided that the foal cannot stick its head through the fence to nurse), but it will take longer this way. If the foal has other foals for company, it will be much happier during the weaning period.

The main problem to avoid at weaning time is injury to foal or dam during their frantic efforts to get back together. This requires safe fencing. Barbed wire, low gates, and rotten boards invite trouble. Occasionally a mare or foal will require tranquilization to ease them through the first day or two of separation.

Many people are overly concerned with the care of the mare during the weaning period. Therefore it helps to understand the physiology of lactation (milk production). Milk is formed by special cells inside the mammary gland, and its raw materials come from the bloodstream. The constant removal of milk encourages the formation of more milk. The actual let-down of milk is stimulated by the foal bumping the udder, and the sensation caused by his nursing, and the warmth of his mouth. When one considers this, it becomes obvious that massage, heat, and milking out the udder is *not* the way to dry up a mare.

Yet when many people see the udder swollen and full of milk soon after the foal is removed, they start milking the mare out, rubbing the udder with camphorated oil, and applying warm packs.

Occasionally a mare or foal will require tranquilization to ease them through the first day or two of separation.

143

Just the reverse should be done. Allow the udder to fill. Once sufficient pressure is established, nature will know that the milk is no longer required and milk secretion will grind to a halt.

Do *not* massage the udder. If it is hot and swollen and seems painful, apply *cold* packs rather than hot packs. Exercise and withholding grain for a week or so will help dry the mare up.

Once in a while a mare that is a very heavy milk producer will develop severe mammary edema at weaning time. The swelling may extend along the abdominal wall and the udder may be so painful that the mare has difficulty in walking.

For such cases, your veterinarian may prescribe drugs that stimulate the excretion of water, and can spectacularly reduce the swelling overnight. Partially milking out such a mare will prolong the drying-up, but it will also make the process less uncomfortable for the mare.

When large numbers of mares and foals are together in a pasture, weaning may be accomplished by another method. Each day, one mare is removed from the pasture. The foals will miss their mother, but the company of the other foals comforts them and soon all of the foals in the pasture will be weaned and closely bonded.

PROFILE: ROBERT M. MILLER

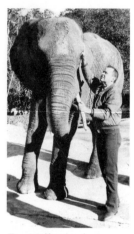

Dr. Miller looks over a patient with unusual conformation.

Except for two years in the Army, I was a student until I was 30 years of age. Summers and weekends I worked with horses (rodeo, wrangler, cowboy, packer, horse breaker). During this time I acquired two degrees: a bachelor's degree in animal science from the University of Arizona (1951) and a doctorate in veterinary medicine from Colorado State University (1956).

I was an Arizona resident and Debby a California resident, but we met at a college rodeo in Colorado and were married in 1956, after we both graduated CSU.

I practiced in Arizona for a year, including some racetrack practice. We then moved to California and founded the Conejo Valley Veterinary Clinic, which grew into an 11-doctor group.

At this writing, our son, Mark, 25, and daughter, Laurel, 19, are both in college.

We have had Quarter Horses since we moved to Thousand Oaks, and have raised quite a few foals. But we got involved with saddle mules in the early 1970s and now have only two broodmares and are currently riding only mules. Debby and Laurel show. Jordass Jean, one of our four mules, was the 1986 world champion performance mule.

My writing and cartooning careers started with *Western Horseman*. I started cartooning for WH before I started vet school and started writing for WH while I was still in vet school.

Besides riding, our main hobby is skiing.

My next book will be on equine behavior.

Distributed to the book trade by
Texas Monthly Press, Inc.
P.O. Box 1569, Austin, TX 78767-1569
Ph. 800-288-3288

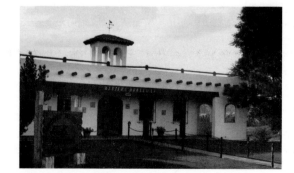

The Western Horseman Magazine, established in 1936, is the world's leading horse publication. For subscription information, write: Western Horseman Magazine, P.O. Box 7980, Colorado Springs, CO 80933-7980.